PEACE
AT
LAST

PEACE
AT
LAST

Stories of Hope and Healing for

Veterans and Their Families

Deborah L. Grassman

Foreword by Daniel R. Tobin, M.D.

VANDAMERE
PRESS

St. Petersburg, Florida

Published by
Vandamere Press
P.O. Box 149
St. Petersburg, FL 33731
USA

Copyright 2009
by Vandamere Press
Second Printing, August 2010
Third Printing, January 2011
Fourth Printing, September 2011
Fifth Printing, February 2012
Sixth Printing, June 2014

ISBN 978-0-918339-72-0

Dedication

*Working at the Department of Veteran's Affairs (VA)
means a life devoted to bringing our soldiers back
home in one piece. The "piece" includes emotional
and spiritual dimensions of self; coming "back home"
may not occur until years after discharge from military
service and is often a long process. Many of my VA
colleagues work tirelessly and unceasingly to restore
wholeness to veterans. This book is dedicated to these
unsung heroes who "serve those who first served us."
They have inspired me. Unsung heroes also include
those many community hospice staff and organizations
who have rallied around this work, recognizing and
supporting the "homecoming" each veteran deserves.
They have humbled me.*

Acknowledgements

Though I am the sole author of this book, it has not been written alone. I've had the support of many people who have encouraged the development of my career and my ideas that have culminated in this book. I cannot possibly cite all of the people whose words, actions, or ideas have impacted me. However, some of the people who have inspired me are cited in the narratives told in this book; it's important to me that they be credited by name. They are: Betty Heffner, R.N., Carol Tripplitt, R.N., Takeshi Okano, M.D., Marie Bainbridge, R.N., Mary Zielinski R.N., Margurite Oliver, Maxine Wehry, Brenda Jackson, R.N., Ursula Hahn, R.Ph., Lorraine Acompora, L.P.N., Dan Hummer, M.Div., John Hull, M.D., Isla Wilburn, L.P.N., Sheila Lozier, R.N., Karina Schwarz, Jim Donahue, and Shirl Swan-Mock, R.N. Most certainly these, and many other staff members not cited here, have been most responsible for my growth and development.

I'm indebted to my supervisors, Christy Galbreath, M.S.N, Joy Easterly, M.S.N., and John Frutchey, M.D. for valuing and supporting this work so some of my clinical responsibilities could be relieved to permit teaching and travel. This book would not have been possible without their insights, efforts, and love for veterans.

I'm also indebted and inspired by the Chief of Home and Community Based Care for the Department of Veterans Affairs in Washington, D.C., Thomas Edes, M.D. His passion for caring for veterans provides the leadership needed for the Department of Veterans Affairs to partner with community hospices so veterans' deaths can be honored. Diane Jones, S.W. (consultant to the VA for developing Hospice-Veterans partnerships) and Scott Shreve, D.O. (Director of Hospice and Palliative Care for the VA) have also been inspirations in providing end-of-life care.

I've been grateful for a group of colleagues who have willingly been readers, editors, and collective-memory keepers with me. We've enjoyed several nights of cheese and chocolate fondues together while I struggled to assimilate and integrate their collective feedback. They've been forced to join me on my journey, providing valued feedback and support in the process. My gratitude is beyond words. They include: Lorraine Acompora, L.P.N, Cookie Baickle, A.R.N.P., Marie Bainbridge, R.N., Ed Chaffin (volunteer), Shaku Desai, R.N., Joanne Flynn, R.N., John Frutchey, M.D., Jennifer Henius, S.W., Brenda Jackson, R.N., Pat Kelley, R.N., Mary Ann Lane, S.W., Pat McGuire, R.N., Jane Sheridan, R.N., Mary Ellen Smith, R.D., Jackie Walsch, A.R.N.P., Mark Walters, Isla Wilburn, L.P.N., and Mary Zielinski, R.N.

Neither do I exempt my family and friends. They have guided my writings to a more meaningful whole. They include: David Grassman, Sarah Grassman, Shannon Grassman, Aaron Grassman, Gail Moore, Sidney Geier, Gail Horsley, Ferol Martin, Suzi Martin, and Cory Raynor.

I also want to acknowledge the hard work of editor Karen Lindsey in helping this manuscript evolve. I'll always be grateful for the many ways she's helped me hone my writing skills. I'm also indebted to Arthur Brown of Vandamere Press for valuing the material in this book. A Vietnam veteran himself, his guidance and insight have been invaluable. Editor, Pat Berger, has also provided important feedback to guide the development of this book.

I'd be remiss if I didn't acknowledge the hard work, support, and insight of Pat McGuire, the Bereavement Coordinator on our unit and Lorraine Acompora. They have been my biggest cheerleaders and have developed into surprisingly effective press agents!

Certainly, the most abiding influence in the development of this work for publication has been Daniel Tobin, M.D., author of *Peaceful Dying*. He has been like a rudder on a sailboat whose skipper didn't always know which port to seek. The only reason this book has materialized is because of Dr. Tobin's unwavering faith in the importance of its message and his love for veterans.

I can only feel gratitude, warmth, and humility in accepting the help of so many generous friends, colleagues, and fellow travelers helping our veterans and each other make the heroic journey home to ourselves.

Table of Contents

Foreword

On a sunny day in the spring of 2004, I drove three hours from our offices in Albany, New York, to the Bronx Veteran's Administration (VA) Medical Center to hear a talk I knew would be important. Deborah Grassman, a nurse practitioner in the Bay Pines, VA Medical Center was speaking on the importance of recognizing the special needs of combat veterans facing advancing illness and end–of-life situations. At the time, I was a consultant to the VA Healthcare Network Upstate New York and was involved in creating health counseling services. I had heard about Deborah and her work, and was anxious to learn more about it. Sitting in the audience listening to Deborah's presentation, I was struck by her passion to tell others about her discoveries. I was moved to tears as I listened to her explain the value of simply thanking veterans for their service and sacrifice. As she went on to discuss her ideas for creating new, focused support services for veterans coping with serious illness, I felt called to service.

My own group, The Center for Advanced Illness Coordinated Care (CAICC), was involved in research and development of evidence-based health counseling, and I saw that we could help Deborah's work get to more veterans. After her talk, I went up and introduced myself. "This is really important," I said to her. "You have to create research to study an intervention and expand the effort with national training programs to further help veterans and their families. And then you have to write a book about it!"

She looked a little startled. Then she smiled. "How do you do that?" she asked.

"I'll help you," I replied. "I've done this sort of thing, and it's less overwhelming than it sounds."

Deborah took me at my word. For the next few years, she dedicated much of her time to creating her ideas and writing this book.

It has been a privilege to have helped her. Deborah has organized some important original concepts within this book, and she has artfully crafted this information into its current form. Veterans, especially combat veterans, need and deserve special services to help them in a preventive as well as supportive manner throughout their lives.

I have worked as a physician health counselor and as a health system administrator and health services researcher. This work has involved helping many veterans face the practical, emotional, and spiritual crises of advanced illness. Throughout all of my work in bringing health care services to veterans, I have been impressed with the way serving in the military and in combat significantly change the individual, especially when facing serious illness. Early on in my career, I spent a great deal of time at the bedside of dying men in the VA Medical Center in Albany, New York, creating programs that helped veterans explore, on the level they were comfortable, issues around finding peace of mind and meaning in reflecting on life. I recall several World War II veterans who requested specific guidance in coming to peace with some of the struggles that *Peace at Last* explores with sensitivity.

Many of the men I worked with had seen death and dying in the brutal, direct processes of war and approached their own serious illness and imminent dying with stoicism. Some needed more help confronting and expressing fears in order to face personal issues. *Peace at Last* presents important information for healthcare providers as well as family members. It will help us all better understand the unique experiences and characters of veterans. Often these are people who have experienced serious trauma and who downplay their suffering. Clearly, combat and battlefield coping can be further complicated by Post Traumatic Stress Disorder (PTSD), which requires special understanding and care. It is helpful to individualize support and services for veterans. This book explores various ways that serious trauma can be integrated into a healthy life.

Each of America's wars has been different in both practical and cultural ways, and it is helpful to analyze our nation's relationship with each era's veterans. It has taken courage for Deborah to travel the country and raise consciousness about the effects that war has on its veterans and the need to refine our approaches to caring for them. As our nation continues to recognize the need for improving access to veteran's benefits of all kinds there is an opportunity for community and government partnership that can redefine our nation's relationship with its veterans. As a country, we can embrace the idea that it is a sign of strength, not weakness, to wholeheartedly welcome veterans home from battle by employing and creating the best services available to care for them in their return.

Recognizing that there are tested and proven methods of addressing the issues of homeless veterans, suicide prevention and PTSD, we need to be rigorous about integrating expanded services throughout the country and about accepting accountability for their outcomes. We have the opportunity and responsibility to learn how to better understand the science of violence and how to integrate prevention and new evidence-based treatments with the human experience of serious trauma. Our freedom and progressive way of life have been fought for by our veterans and their families. As a grateful nation that honors the bond between soldiers and resiliency within the human spirit, we have to be certain that we meet the daily ongoing needs of our veterans in a timely and effective manner.

Inspiration for achieving success in joining community and government organizations to serve our veterans can be drawn from the author, Walter Lord, whose quote is etched in the World War II memorial in Washington, D.C. It states, "Even against the greatest of odds, there is something in the human spirit—a magic blend of skill, faith and valor—that can lift men from certain defeat to incredible victory."

Dan Tobin
Albany, New York

Preface

"**I** could never do what you do!" I hear this exclamation often from people when they find out I'm a Hospice nurse at the Department of Veterans Affairs (VA). "Isn't it depressing?" usually follows. I used to think the same way. No one told me I could find peace, joy, and fulfillment in caring for people at the end of their lives. Because I feared death, these secrets remained obscure. Neither did anyone tell me about caring for veterans. I had no reason to think that veterans' needs were any different from nonveterans. Now I know differently. Certainly I never anticipated that I would learn lessons about peace from people who were trained for war. Warriors often have wisdom that, paradoxically, shows us how to live in peace—with each other and within ourselves.

I have gathered these stories while caring for thousands of veterans over a 25-year career. The selection of stories is biased because it reflects only those veterans who have received care at the VA, which is about 15% of the veteran population. Each story offers insights that may or may not be applicable to the broader veteran population.

It's not easy to decide which stories to tell in this book. Some stories may have been more relevant to tell, but made less of an impact on me personally so I can't tell them as authentically. For example, you won't hear stories like the schizophrenic patient who lay dying without family. When I came into the room, his psychiatrist was kneeling at his side and with tears in her eyes, said, "He lived like a pauper, but he's dying like a king." I don't know that patient's story, but I suspect if I asked that physician, she would tell me a story worth beholding.

The stories that didn't make the book are no less important; they are stories written on my soul rather than these pages. For this reason, I've included my own personal musings that describe how I've let "warrior wisdom" change and inspire me. So join me in a journey that is not often told, to discover hidden worlds of nurses, traumatized victims, dying people, and veteran culture. You might be surprised at what you discover.

Chapter One

Rescuing the World
from Suffering

I was intent on rescuing the world from suffering
not realizing my idealistic mission
was like saving fish from drowning.
It would take years of listening to patients
before I realized they weren't drowning
and what they really needed was for me to learn how to swim.
The problem was
I thought I already knew how.[1]

I had always been squeamish at the sight of gore and passed out at
the sight of blood. This didn't bode well for a young woman wanting a career as a nurse. Then it occurred to me I could acclimate
myself to blood and guts by practicing on fish I caught from the Gulf
of Mexico. I set upon my mission feeling like the locomotive in *The
Little Engine that Could.* Through squinted eyes and gritted teeth,
turning my head away as far as I could while still spying the incision
site, touching the fish with just the ends of my thumb and forefin-
ger to minimize contact with its disgusting slime, I inserted a knife
into the limp belly and hesitantly slit it open. I actually retched when
I reached in to grab the entrails, tugging and tearing them free from
their attachments.

"You can do this Deborah. If you want to become a nurse, you
will do this," I kept determinedly repeating to myself, and 50 or 60
fish later, I did.

At the time, I didn't recognize the importance of that decision.
Now, I look back on the moment recognizing its significance, grateful I had the "guts" to face guts, grateful I was willing to suffer my
retching and overwhelming desire for escape. It has been an impor-

tant asset for what would become my life's work in an unanticipated environment for patients I had no anticipated desire to serve.

Entering a Different World

I was a student nurse interning my way through numerous hospitals. Rotations at the Department of Veterans Affairs (VA) hospital were different from civilian medical centers. It started at the entrance. A sign proclaimed: "The Price of Freedom Is Visible Here." A gate protected access. Entering the VA hospital in Saint Petersburg, Florida, was like passing into an alternate dimension where new realities and time warps were juxtaposed against ordinary activities of daily living.

Other hospitals I had rotated through had female patients; other hospitals had private and semiprivate rooms. At Bay Pines VA Medical Center, female patients were seldom seen and most private rooms were replaced with twelve-bed wards. There was no mistaking the military décor either: green walls, green tile floors, green hallways, green gastric contents in the portable Gomco suction machines at the bedsides. Only those few patients who were lucky enough to be near an uncurtained window were provided green relief.

As drab and monotonous as the interior was, the exterior was colorful and interesting. Spanish stucco buildings stood majestic with colorful intricate tiles over Mediterranean Revival doorways, windows, and porticoes. "Progress" loomed in the background. A new modern-looking hospital with a monotonous government facade was incongruously intermingled with the historical architecture, corrupting the landscape with disharmony.

The entrances were unique to the VA hospital as well. During most hours of the day, a conclave of wheel-chaired patients "stood guard" (or I should say "sat guard"), elbows on armrests, shoulders hunched and leaning forward with heads hung, cigarettes in hand (often rough, yellowed hands), swapping military stories. Student nurses passing by were ogled, but usually with respect (probably because of our uniforms).

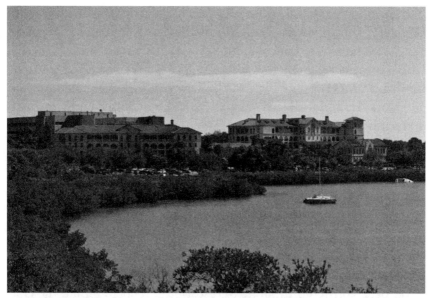

Original Spanish buildings at Bay Pines VA Medical Center.[2]

VA Photograph

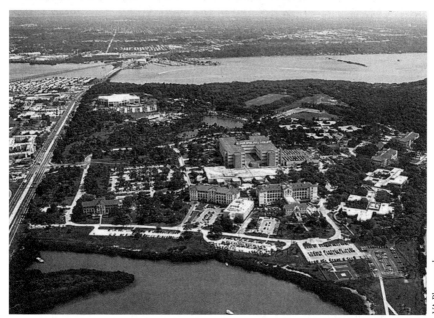

Aerial view of Bay Pines surrounded by Boca Ciega Bay with newer contemporary buildings shown in center.

VA Photograph

Beyond the buildings lay tall pines, a serene oak-lined military cemetery, and the bejeweled Gulf of Mexico. While other hospitals were surrounded by concrete, an occasional sparrow, and the everywhere-present squirrel, the spacious 337 acres of the VA grounds were surrounded by rabbits, turtles, armadillos, eagles, herons, and alligators. In a Florida city congested with condominiums, tourists, and traffic, the VA hospital was like a surprising calm in the center of a tumultuous hurricane.

Bay Pines was its own city within the city of St. Petersburg, with its own post office and zip code. It had its own federal police force. It was self-contained—literally. In the event of a national emergency, this VA could sustain itself for 30 days without outside water, electricity, or supplies. Bay Pines had a history, too. It was rumored that the property had been confiscated by the federal government from gangster, Al Capone, for failure to pay income taxes (though I've never been able to corroborate that story). Long before that, the land had been a sacred burial ground for Timucuan Indians who occupied the land between 1,000 BC and 1,500 AD.[3] Today, Bay Pines is listed on the National Historical Register.

To a student nurse unused to VA hospitals, it wasn't just a new city, it was a whole new world. My first patient was in his early 50s, admitted for evaluation of abdominal pain. Our assignment was to practice our newly acquired bed-making and bed-bath skills. We had been instructed to make crisp corners with bed linens and maintain proper privacy and dignity while providing hygiene to the patients' private areas. Though capable of providing his own hygiene, this patient graciously obliged my need for a learning experience. I dawdled with the wash cloth in the basin of water figuring out how to approach his private parts without betraying my embarrassment, mentally practicing how to do it matter-of-factly as if I did this all the time. I don't recall how well I was able to disguise my ineptitude, but what I do recall is the instructor's look when she peeped around the curtains to see how I was doing. I finished up and trotted over to see what she wanted.

"For those patients who are able, you can just give them a warm washcloth and let them clean their own genitalia," she whispered.

"Oh," I said, feeling foolish. The smile on the guy's face and twinkle in his eye now took on a whole new meaning!

On another occasion, I answered a call light. The patient asked me for a "duck."

"A what?" I asked incredulously.

"A duck."

Not seeing any feathers or hearing any quacking, I thought he was playing a joke on me. "I don't think duck is on the menu today."

"You know. A urinal. Can you give me a urinal?"

I burst out laughing. I had just been indoctrinated into military lingo, discovering that evidently the shape of the older, white-enameled urinals reminded soldiers of ducks. Thereafter, whenever a patient asked for a duck, I delivered it quacking.

Veterans, I was learning, were not your average patients; neither were the VA nurses caring for them. I remember the night nurse who challenged me to look, listen to, and love aging soldiers. Gruff, square-shouldered, and with 40 years of nursing experience, Betty first greeted me when I came bouncing down the hall at midnight by putting her arm around me stiffly before letting me know what was to come. "All right, Grassman, now I'm going to show you what nursing is *really* about." I gulped, expressed my appreciation, and decided to trust this woman who was willing to share her years of experience with someone so inexperienced.

Two of the first lessons I learned were to whisper and carry a good flashlight. Even my shoes were too loud, thunderously echoing down silent hallways.

"These men are sick, Grassman. They don't sleep well. See to it you change those shoes and don't be turning on those overbed lights unless it's an emergency. These patients need their rest. They don't need the likes of us disturbing them with our carelessness."

I came to realize that as rough as Betty may have sounded, her motives were pure; she wanted to care for and protect her veterans. I listened carefully.

"They've seen things in war you don't want to know about," she told me one day. "Too horrible for them to even talk about; but if they ever say anything, make sure you listen."

I nodded like I already understood, disguising how I'd never even considered that these patients were veterans with a common military history that would impact my care for them. I sensed that these guys needed something more than usual nursing care, but I didn't yet know what it was.

This hospital had a lot of things other hospitals did not, though I was too young and inexperienced to know or care what it was. For now, all I cared about was passing through these VA walls for a required learning experience on my way to becoming a labor and delivery nurse.

The semesters passed, and I did other rotations. Graduation was approaching; employment decisions needed to be made. I found that my aspiration for maternity nursing was gradually eroding. Instead, I was thinking about the VA hospital. In my final rotation there, I asked my nurse mentors why they had chosen to work at the VA. Each had their own, unique reasons:

"I came because I had a neighbor who was a bilateral amputee from the Korean War. He worked as a nursing assistant at the VA. I never forgot that."

"I came because I was a member of the Cooties (an honor organization of the Veterans of Foreign Wars who provide service to veterans). It seemed natural to work here."

"I'm a veteran. Coming here to work was like coming home. It didn't seem much different than what I was used to. I can transfer from one VA to the other, anywhere in the country. My years in the military count toward my retirement, too."

"My father taught me to be patriotic—like standing up when the flag passed. He encouraged me to work here so I could take care of veterans."

These unique reasons contrasted with nurses who worked in community hospitals. Aside from their dedication to a difficult profession, their decisions about where to work were usually based on location, convenience, or wages. While this was perfectly reasonable, it lacked the intrigue that the VA nurses had provided. I didn't know what kind of nursing I wanted to do, but I now knew where I wanted to do it.

"Why in the world would you want to work for the VA?" a classmate asked. "It's so drab and dreary there. All you're going to do is care for old men." I had clearly picked an unpopular area for nursing; indeed, I was the only student in my graduating class of 250 who came to work for the VA.

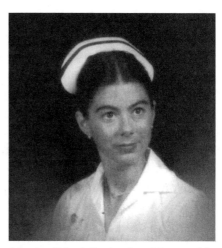

Nursing School Graduation: 31 years old.

"These guys are hard to love," I told her loftily. "But I can do it. They need my love," I told her.

In addition to thinking that veterans needed to be loved, I was thinking about Florence Nightingale. She had founded nursing while serving soldiers in the Crimean War. I felt a kinship to this first "VA" nurse. Reading her biography helped me realize how passion, persistence, and keen observation can create systems and environments that respond to veterans' needs. She had learned these lessons in large wards filled with war-weary soldiers. I decided I could do the same, but it wasn't as simple as I initially imagined. Though I had sensed the brokenness in some of these veterans' hardened souls, I was arrogant and naïve; I thought I was the person who could fix them. It would take years of chipping away at my seemingly altruistic façade before I realized just how little I understood, and it never occurred to me to ask what sometimes made them so hard to love.

A Registered Nurse at Last

At last, spring of 1983 arrived and I graduated. I felt proud to finally be able to don my white hat and write the coveted initials "R.N."

after my name; I didn't feel like a nurse on the inside, though. I walked each day from the parking lot, through the path under the towering pine trees, praying, "God, please don't let me kill anyone today." One day, I thought I did. I walked onto the ward and was instantly confronted by a nurse swinging an IV bag back and forth in front of me.

"Know what this is?" she asked jeeringly. When I shook my head, she went on. "It's $D_5 1/2$ normal saline that you hung. It should have been $D_5 1/4$ normal saline."

I hung my head as she showed me the incident report she had completed, feeling the shame she intended for me. Though I didn't realize it then, I was being indoctrinated into the nursing culture. Later when I heard that "nurses eat their young," I knew what it meant.

I saw the errant IV bag and the incident report lying on my head nurse's desk all day. The head nurse, Carol, saw me pass her office several times, yet said nothing. Nearing the end of shift, I could stand it no longer. I poked my head into Carol's office and hesitantly asked her if she wanted to see me about the medication error I had made.

"No, Deborah, I don't," she said. I looked at her without understanding. "I know you well enough to know that you learn from your mistakes. There's nothing I can say that you haven't already said to yourself."

I stood there dumbfounded. Then she matter-of-factly dismissed me to go on about my work. She taught me something *beyond* careful medication administration; she taught me that it was okay to make a mistake as long as I learned from it.

I also recall my first hurricane as a nurse. My husband, children, and I had evacuated to a friend's house. Most hurricanes pass in one day, so I had only taken one change of clothing. However, Hurricane Elena remained off shore for three days, and I was without uniform and accompanying work apparel. My friend was a nurse, so I borrowed her uniform. My 9-year-old son's feet were the same size as mine, so I wore his white tennis shoes and my daughter's soccer socks. My husband had clean underwear; I was surprised at how comfortable they were! We all had a good laugh at getting Mom ready for work. When I went to work, everyone assumed that everything I had on was mine . . . until later that day.

I was kneeling on a patient's bed doing chest compressions after his heart had stopped. In that position, my pant legs rode up revealing the bright red stripes on the top of my daughter's socks and my son's tennis shoes. After the confusion from the emergency was over, the supervisor commented on my footwear.

"Oh. These are my son's shoes and my daughter's socks. And I'm wearing my husband's underwear . . . if you really want to know."

She laughed and added, "I just feel lucky you showed up for work at all today."

"I just feel lucky I have 'one body that fits all'," I retorted.

Laughter was a good way to relax after the tense situation we'd been managing. Code blues (situations in which a person's heart and respirations stop, requiring resuscitation) were frantic, confusing, and exciting. I was slowly growing in expertise so I was less intimidated and more competent in emergency situations. Nurse Betty had taught me about those too. After returning from hastily handling one such situation, Betty had cocked her head to one side, squinted one eye slightly, and in her cigarette-induced gravelly voice said, "You know, Grassman, there's hardly any situation, even emergencies, that wouldn't benefit from taking five seconds to *refrain* from action and instead *think*."

Her advice became one of the cornerstones of my practice.

With increased confidence, I developed ambitions to become an intensive care unit (ICU) nurse. I was enthralled by the machines, lines, and technology. I admired the skill required to manage these competencies. "That's what *real* nurses do. ICU nurses have to be able to do it *all*," I told myself. I promptly enrolled in a course to learn how to read heart monitors.

I don't know if it was naiveté or denial that kept me from remembering that I wasn't particularly mechanically-minded or dexterous. I remember being surprised one day when I overheard a nurse reporting that a patient was a "hard stick" (poor veins that make IV access difficult). The other nurse had replied, "Tell Deborah. She's a good stick." I silently chuckled. I had earned an undeserved title, yet not without merit. Because I was actually a "bad stick," I became very good at finding veins no one else could find that could then be accessed. I was slowly learning that patiently looking for what others are too busy to see was a highly useful skill.

Though I was set on becoming an ICU nurse, other ideas began to occur to me after awhile. It was a stroke patient whose condition started deteriorating that opened my mind to non-ICU possibilities. When his wife came, I told her what had happened. She began softly crying, telling me she knew he was going to die. I don't remember what was said, but I do remember experiencing the sacredness of the moment as she reckoned with the loss and mounted the courage to face letting him go. I remember walking down the hall after leaving her and feeling part of a mystery that was deeper and more powerful than I understood. I also recalled a passage I had read in a book a few years earlier that had made an indelible impact on me: "You are as dead now, as you are ever going to be."

That sentence came back to me in a wave of emotion as I dealt with this patient's death. I hadn't completely understood it then, but sitting at a nurses' station years later, I found myself contemplating this idea that my current form might be more limiting and confining than my future forms. I glimpsed an understanding of the mystery of death that intrigued me even more now than it had when I first read it years earlier.

After a year on the neurology and rehab unit, my supervisor told me she wanted me to transfer to the surgical unit to gain more experience. Though I was still somewhat tied to the idea of eventually working ICU, I liked the idea of doing surgical nursing. Like ICU, surgical nursing with its tubes and technicalities reinforced my idea of what "real" nurses did. I learned a new world of preoperative check lists, chest tubes, and the need to monitor patients for post-surgical complications. This last nursing task could be quite challenging. As the effects of anesthesia wore off, a few of the patients experienced vivid combat memories and became agitated. Sometimes they mistook nurses for enemy soldiers or they thought loud sounds were bombs. Military experience even affected preoperative preparation. One patient was to have a lung removed by a Japanese surgeon, Dr. Okano. As I was explaining the consent form, the patient said, "I know this is irrational. I know the doctor is a good surgeon, but I fought in World War II in the Pacific and I just can't surrender myself to a Japanese man standing over my heart with a knife while I'm asleep."

I hesitantly phoned Dr. Okano to let him know the patient's concerns and to reassure him that it wasn't a question of racism. Luckily, he understood. "It's okay. I've heard this before," he said. "Tell him not to worry. I'll have someone else do the surgery."

I appreciated the wisdom of that surgeon, and I've often wondered how my patient's post-operative recovery might have been complicated if Dr. Okano had not responded so astutely or had taken the patient's fears personally.

With all the skills and tasks required to provide nursing care to surgical patients, putting down naso-gastric tubes was really the only task at which I was able to excel. I'd taught yoga earlier in my life, and this helped me teach patients to relax so I could slip a tube down their noses into their stomachs quickly and easily, even in resistant patients. But I was at best mediocre in other technical skills; I was forced into the realization that my expertise might lie outside both surgical and ICU nursing.

I decided that "real nursing" could also include nontechnical skills that might better suit my abilities. Evidently my supervisor thought so too because she asked me if I would consider a transfer to a medical unit. She said that my eagerness to learn, patient-teaching abilities, and identifying and confronting administrative problems that interfered with patient care were valued by the administration. In fact, they wanted me to consider a leadership position after I gained more clinical experience.

I enjoyed the medical unit, and it was there that my clinical skills finally gelled. I no longer begged God not to let me kill anyone and, in fact, was reasonably confident I could actually help most patients most of the time. However, I remained feeling helpless and ineffective with dying patients and their families. I was afraid of saying the wrong thing. I had not yet personally experienced the death of anyone close to me that might have helped me to understand the needs of the dying. In my middle 30s, I was in the summer of my life, focused on having, gaining, and achieving. Changing, losing, and letting go were not yet my season. Nevertheless, I was fascinated with death.

"I would like a transfer to the oncology unit," I told my supervisor one day. She said she would consider it. A few months later, she brought up the subject again and offered me the Head Nurse position on the oncology unit. I was shocked. Though it was flattering, I was aware of how little I knew about cancer. "Oh no! I can't," I blurted out. "I just want to be a staff nurse."

"Why don't you think about it for a few days?" She asked in a gentle, firm tone. Fearful that I wouldn't be able to transfer to oncology unless I accepted the position, I hesitantly agreed.

I came to the oncology unit timid and intimidated. Every nurse there was at least 10 years my senior, and they all had a wealth of oncology experience I didn't have. (And I was supposed to manage them!) Luckily for me, the oncology nurses were both generous and gracious, taking me under their wings and teaching me what I needed to know.

Oncology was a specialty that contained multiple, complex subspecialties that seemed overwhelming to the neophyte that I was. I soon learned to respect the sophistication and complexities that skilled oncology nursing care required. First, I focused on the intricacies of cancer and its treatment. I learned about chemotherapy drugs and their side effects. I learned about oncology emergencies, blood disorders, and pain management.

It was the nonphysical dimensions of cancer that puzzled and confused me, especially the "negative" feelings of anger, fear, and sadness that often accompany the diagnosis and treatment of cancer. Initially, I felt helpless, inadequate, and ineffective in responding to patients or families in these difficult situations. Rather than experience these feelings, I tried to control them by avoiding the emotional aspects of the illness. I also tried to control veterans' feelings of loss by encouraging them to focus on the bright side. I even designed teaching programs to help them stay positive about their experience. Some of the classes helped people manage side effects; others dealt with the emotional and spiritual distress that the disease caused. I used videotapes and books designed for cancer patients. Most had themes of encouragement like: "You can do it," "Hang in there," "Keep fighting," "Think positively," "Chemo is your friend," "Focus on the 50% who survive this disease." I made posters for the unit with similar themes. The messages were essentially: "What you are going through is not as bad as it seems," "There is always hope for recovery," "Maintain a good attitude and do these things and you can control what is happening to you."

Some of these efforts helped our veterans deal with their illness. Others only encouraged their grin-and-bear-it attitudes; their suffering became silent so that the rest of us would not have to be touched by their distress. Yet, no matter what we did, most of our patients had progressive disease that was beyond surgical or radiological intervention when they were diagnosed; chemotherapeutic cures were rare at that time.

I'm not sure when I started questioning the impact our messages of "fight," "hope," and "control" might be having on those patients who fought, hoped, and tried to control what was ultimately beyond control. Were we multiplying their suffering? Were we reinforcing denial? Were we doing these things to make ourselves feel less helpless and more in control? While we were teaching patients what and how to control, what were we doing to teach them how to deal with their loss of control? While we were telling them that they need not suffer, what *were* we doing to validate the suffering they *were* feeling? Though all the things we were teaching were true, perhaps we were creating half-truths by not acknowledging, discussing, and preparing patients for how to let go when the time comes when they will not survive.

We had carefully followed American Cancer Society guidelines. Our program was even professionally recognized and published in an oncology journal,[4] but perhaps our perspectives simply reflected the larger medical culture. I decided to adopt a different tactic: let my patients teach me what they needed. I started listening to them more carefully; I wanted to hear what they were saying and, just as importantly, to what they were *not* saying. I refrained from speaking so intensely or giving advice so matter-of-factly. I stopped trying to rescue patients from their feelings of anger, fear, pain, guilt, loneliness, helplessness, and uncertainty they were trying to express. I let go of the need to control my own fear of helplessness and inadequacy and instead let myself experience these feelings.

Repeatedly, patients showed me that rather than having me try to minimize their emotional suffering, they needed to have it validated. They helped me see how much loss they were experiencing and how much support they needed to manage the changes they were going through.

The more our oncology team acknowledged and listened to patients' difficulties, the more we became convinced of their need for medical professionals who were trained in hospice and palliative care.[5] While it made sense to focus on recovery skills when recovery was still feasible, it didn't mean that we couldn't also include techniques for helping them face the time when they would not recover. That way, they would be ready for anything that happened. As we started openly including ways to emotionally and spiritually prepare for the end of life, patients reported they felt better. Many reported that, paradoxically, letting go of the fear of death helped them experience life more fully.

In response to this need, our hospital administration approved funding for a 10-bed Hospice and Palliative Care unit. One section of the oncology unit was modified to create a homelike environment. A living room, kitchen, and chapel were added. Sofas opened into beds so families could remain close. Unrestricted visiting hours and pet visitation contributed to a soft environment. Carpeted hallways, peaceful music, and incandescent lighting created soothing ambience.

I became the clinician who screened patients for admission to the Hospice and Palliative Care program. I also provided consultation to patients throughout the hospital on how to face serious illness. I thought few adjustments would be needed to expand services to include hospice and palliative care. I thought this would simply be an extension of what we had already learned about providing pain relief and symptom management. I was wrong. I hadn't considered that I knew our oncology patients well because I had nursed them through treatment and complications for many months prior to their deaths. As oncology staff, we had time to develop relationships with them. We had time to discover the meaning in their lives gradually, and to support them incrementally as they neared the ends of their lives. This was not the case with our hospice patients. They arrived on our doorsteps strangers—dying strangers—often with just a few days or weeks to live. We no longer had the luxury of time. Out of the 275 patients we cared for each year, 40 percent died within 48 hours. We had to learn how to develop relationships quickly and respond to their physical, emotional, and spiritual needs promptly.

To enhance my expertise, I went to graduate school to pursue a Master's degree in psychiatric nursing. It provided an opportunity to learn more about nonphysical aspects of oncology and hospice care. My internships were designed to learn the intricacies in providing emotional and spiritual support. It wasn't educational degrees or internships, however, that taught me what I needed to know in order to care for veterans; it was the veterans themselves. One after another, they chipped away at what I thought I knew and taught me what I needed to know. They showed me what set them apart from non-veterans. They also showed me how my own attitudinal barriers kept me distant from them. It was a crucial lesson.

Initial Lessons

- Develop guts.
- Let go of what you think you know and open up to what others have to teach you.
- Stay open to your mistakes so you can learn from them.
- Laughter brings perspective.
- Refrain from acting hastily and instead *think*.
- Patiently watch for things you'd otherwise be too busy to see.
- Challenge your own thinking.
- Remember that you're as dead now as you're ever going to be.
- Not acknowledging the possibility of failure is a half-truth that robs people of the opportunity to learn how to come to peace with limitations.
- Stop trying to rescue people from their feelings of anger, fear, pain, guilt, loneliness, helplessness, and uncertainty that they experience. Instead, open up to their feelings and experience them too. Validate their suffering.
- Let go of the need to control your own fear of helplessness and inadequacy and instead let yourself become vulnerable by experiencing these feelings.
- Including ways to emotionally and spiritually prepare for the end of life, paradoxically, helps people experience life more fully.

Chapter Two

A Reluctant Witness

He jests at scars
who never felt a wound.
—Shakespeare[1]

He had fractured his clavicle by simply turning his head. Later, he similarly fractured his arm. Fred had weakened bones throughout his cancer-riddled skeleton. Despite these hardships, his wife, Peggy, managed his care at home, driving him 100 miles to the VA Medical Center for monthly treatments.

One time Fred had to be hospitalized. We were helping him move to a bedside commode when his thigh bone broke. Howling in pain, he shifted his weight to the other leg. In an instant, his hip broke too. Peggy heard the bones snap and was beside herself. I took her out of the room while staff worked to stabilize his fractures.

"This is so unfair," I told Peggy tearfully.

I could see Peggy took comfort in these words as I validated the suffering she was feeling.

"I don't know what we've done to deserve this," she said softly. She cried for awhile then shook herself to regain her composure. Having confronted her own feelings, she was now able to return to the room to comfort Fred.

A few days later, the staff needed to use a mechanical lift to raise Fred from the bed so a special mattress could be placed under him. We knew this would be excruciating for him, but Fred refused any pain medication; all I could do was shut the door and tell him to scream or do whatever he needed to help his distress. However, Fred had been a soldier in World War II. He knew what it took to survive, and the way soldiers survive is through sheer grit and determination.

He never made a sound. While held aloft in the lift, gritting his teeth as if biting a bullet, face knotted tightly in pain, he winked at me. "How ya doin' Deb?"

I was stunned by his stoicism. Though I had seen it with hundreds of other veterans, it was as if I were seeing it for the first time. Rather than focus on their own pain, they focused on others. They could be wincing in pain and yet when asked, reply "I can handle it" or "It's just a little discomfort." For some, the more pain the better; it was proof of how strong they were. "Breaking down" to take pain medication signified failure. The military magnified the "big boys don't cry" attitudes already instilled in little boys; male soldiers received a double dose of "macho."

Fred died a few days later, never complaining. His face remained taut until the last hours of life when stoicism finally yielded to the peace and freedom of death. I was haunted by his determination not to succumb to what he was experiencing, to fight until the bitter end.

Fred remained on my mind. I realized I had often admired the stoicism I witnessed in so many veterans. They were uncomplaining, "grin and bear it" types, who endured their sufferings silently. The few times tears or fears broke through their façades, they felt embarrassed; they apologized, and quickly re-retreated. Walls offered protection. Yet, I noted their "fight-to-the-bitter-end" attitudes sometimes meant just that: fighting to deaths that were indeed bitter. "Attack and defend" instincts made death the enemy and dying a battle. Survival mode mentality interfered with letting go. When backed into a corner, soldiers weren't conditioned to surrender; they were conditioned to fight.

I had never attempted to broach, much less breach, stoic façades; something in Fred's eyes during those last three days made me question my wisdom in failing to do so. Was his stoicism such a good thing after all? What purpose had it served Fred and other veterans like him? I began to wonder if it was really an unqualified virtue after all. Could stoicism contribute to the agitation and lack of peace I sometimes witnessed as veterans died? While I was busy praising veterans for being "good patients" because they seldom cried, complained of pain, or spoke of fear, was I reinforcing facades that might be detrimental to their well-being? While I was reinforcing the façade, was I missing an opportunity to help them learn how to let go? Would they be less able to face and accept death peacefully because of their "don't surrender" training?

Marie, one of our Hospice nurses, confirmed my suspicions. "How much pain do you need to die?" she asked me exasperatedly one day. She was frustrated by the stoicism she was witnessing with a patient who kept refusing pain medication in spite of his suffering. This attitude may have served him well years ago on the battlefield, but what happens when he's no longer a soldier and needs to confront life as a husband, a father, or a dying human being?

Then I realized that one of the reasons for my admiration of veterans' stoicism was caused by fear of my own emotions. I had often erected a stoic wall to "fight/flight/freeze" emotional pain; I pretended all was well, foolishly hiding feelings from myself and others. Whenever a lump came to my throat, it was shoved down along with the embarrassing tears that brought it forth. I suddenly remembered a moment from my childhood when I tearfully watched the TV show Lassie. Lassie's 6-year-old owner was in danger, and the collie was coming to his rescue. When my Dad walked in the room and saw me crying, he laughed. In my 5-year-old mind, I decided I would never give him any tears to laugh about again; and I didn't. Thirty years later, my childhood decision was still exerting its influence.

I also realized I used denial to deal with many of my personal problems. Rather than let myself feel emotional pain or inadequacy, I either pretended I didn't have a problem or minimized problems by saying, "It's no big deal." I realized that years of seeing my parents' belittling response to overt emotion had sent my feelings underground. I created a calm, cool veneer. Like a callus formed to prevent sensitive blisters, it spared my parents having to deal with my feelings; now I didn't know how to deal with them either.

I made a decision not to let myself miss or anesthetize whatever pain I was feeling. It was a good decision, but it wasn't easy to implement initially. In fact, I reverted to my previous avoidance behaviors. This reaction isn't really surprising considering how close I was to the patient. Dave had cancer of the head and neck and had undergone a laryngectomy, breathing through a hole made in his throat. Besides having chemo treatments five days each month on our unit, Dave worked 40 hours a week as a volunteer for us. As a retired engineer, he was highly efficient, and our whole unit depended on him. After about a year, his condition began to deteriorate, and he was admitted with weakness and shortness of breath.

"I'm going to die in two weeks," he announced one day.

I visited him whenever I could during the next week and we talked about everything, everything, that is, except his approaching death. The following week, I didn't get to his room as much. "I'm too busy," I told myself.

True to his word, Dave was dying at the end of two weeks. Called to his room, I watched helplessly. After he died and everyone left, I prepared his body for the morgue. The pain I'd denied and the tears I had held back came rushing forth. Dave wasn't just another patient. He'd been my friend and coworker for more than a year. He'd been through rough times and I'd always been there for him, up until his last week.

For the next few weeks, I ran from my grief and guilt. My usual ability to dismiss a distressing thought didn't seem to work. I could feel the blocked energy. I realized my fear of pain might be worse than the pain itself. I decided to abide my grief and reckon with the pain. In addition to the guilt I felt about abandoning Dave, I hurt with the realization that I had missed the opportunity to tell him what he had meant to me and thank him for the service he had provided our unit.

I held a staff meeting to discuss the needs of dying patients. I shared my feelings about Dave's death and how I'd avoided him, denying us both the chance to say good-bye. Other staff shared similar feelings. Publicly, I asked Dave for forgiveness. "I'm sorry for not being there when you needed me. I'm sorry my fear kept me away. Because of you, I now commit to letting go of my cowardice so that other patients won't have to die alone."

Through all the tears and the guilt of letting down a friend, there also came the beginning of healing. I realized it had only come when I'd let myself acknowledge the pain and share it with others. That meeting started a monthly tradition of our team coming together to share our vulnerabilities and connections. It proved invaluable for our individual and collective growth.

The first chance to put my renewed determination to practice came with Larry, a 43-year-old with recurrent lung cancer who had frequent hospitalizations. As his condition declined, he became intermittently disoriented. During a confused moment, he asked me to shave him. As I did, he became focused, looking into my eyes.

"Am I dying?" he asked.

I nodded slowly not deflecting my gaze from his. "It's possible," I told him gently.

I remembered my commitment to Dave and began to tell Larry how much he meant to me. He told me how comforting I'd been to him. He added that he was ready to die and thanked me for talking with him about it. When Larry died a few days later, my grief was mixed with a deep satisfaction and peace.

I still got scared and wanted to withdraw emotionally so I could flight pain, but as I felt this impulse, I began talking to myself to provide en-courage-ment: "It's okay to hurt. It's okay to feel what you feel. You gotta *feel* life as well as think about it. Breathe and feel, Deborah. Breathe and feel . . . "

Little by little, I experienced healing from the emotional wounds caused by suppressed pain. I was learning how to let myself feel all of life, including its sorrows. I was starting to understand the axiom, "You can't heal what you don't feel."

Anger was the next feeling I dared to feel. It's the one exception of feelings that is sanctioned for boys. Big boys aren't supposed to cry, but it's okay for them to stomp their feet. Feeling angry is more comfortable than feeling pain for most men in American culture. Anger wards off feelings of vulnerability and helplessness. Furthermore, it often discourages self-awareness, focusing blame on others. In military systems, anger is one of the few feelings that is authorized; it mobilizes soldiers to conquer and control. Working with veterans, I was beginning to see how anger mobilized people to attack or defend.

I also knew anger caused stress hormones like adrenalin to rise and that adrenalin caused responses that are often referred to as fighting or flighting. If emotional pain is experienced as a threat to well-being, the pain is "flighted" with alcohol, television, and other distractions or addictions. On the other hand, anger can *fight* emotional pain. Anger keeps the hurt away. Hurt makes us feel vulnerable and helpless; anger can make us feel strong and powerful. Alternatively, we might feel overwhelmed by the stressor, *freezing* in anxiety and immobilized by a sense of helplessness. Frozen, the stoic wall can become thicker.

For little girls, it's usually the opposite. "Good girls don't get angry." Displays of anger bring disapproval, thwarting desires to please and be accepted. Just as many men put pain at a distance with anger, many women keep anger at a distance with emotional pain; tears are more acceptable in women. They can even feel guilty for having angry feelings or that their anger causes others to feel unhappy. Feeling hurt becomes more comfortable and natural than feeling angry. Some of us, myself included, get two for the price of one; we learn to suppress both anger and pain. Having learned how to touch and feel my pain, I knew my next journey needed to be experiencing and feeling my anger. A patient showed me how little I knew. It happened when I went into his room, inviting him to attend our emotional support group we have for patients.

"I don't want to go to any God-damn meeting," he yelled, glaring. "I just want the results of my biopsy. Can't anyone around here tell me whether or not I have cancer?"

I was stunned. "You don't have to yell at me," I said coldly. "You can just tell me how you feel." Indignantly, I walked out of the room and promptly asked the psychologist to come deal with this patient's "inappropriate" behavior. That evening, I recalled how uncomfortable I was with the patient's anger and how justified I had felt in defending myself. Then I realized his anger was normal and healthy, and it was my response that was askew. Intimidated by his anger, I had failed to address its cause or help to expedite his biopsy results. I had blamed him for feeling as he did, rather than responding to his frustration at not getting vital information.

Once again, I made a commitment; this time I'd stop feeling threatened by anger and instead learn from it. "I want to feel all of myself. Open me to my anger. Help me see and feel what I don't want to see and feel," I prayed.

A patient named Don soon tested my resolution. Only 32 years old, he had recurrent testicular cancer, and he was furious about it. Abusive and difficult, he'd alienated nurses and threatened to stop treatment. I was called to his room to mediate a tense standoff between him and Sally, one of the nurses. Don was nearly 7-feet tall, and I'm only 5 feet, but I sent everyone away, promising myself I wouldn't be intimidated by his anger.

Don ranted and raved, calling the nurse a "fuckin' bitch." Normally I would have taken offense at such abuse and defended my staff, but this time, I decided I would just listen before I determined what stand I would take.

Soon Don started yelling about how he resented losing control of his life: his plans, his ability to work, his ability to have sex. Though I was intimidated by his anger, I remained resolute to hear it so I could discover its source.

"Could it be your cancer that's the 'fuckin' bitch'?" I asked quietly.

He started sobbing, telling me how scared he was and how he grieved for his life. In allowing him his anger, I had helped him see through it to the pain underneath. Finally he looked up and asked, "Why can't I quit crying?"

"Because you have a lot of uncried tears," I told him. "All your plans have been snatched away. Of course you're angry. You have a lot to cry about with all these changes in your life. Let yourself feel your pain, Don. Then you'll find a better way to live with all that's happened."

His suffering validated, he reached out and hugged me. He went out to find Sally. He apologized and hugged her; they both cried together.

I was amazed that healing could be on the other side of such anger. I was surprised to discover how anger masked pain. I also realized that just as I'd masked my own pain, I'd also hidden from my anger. To me, anger was a negative feeling well-adjusted people didn't have. I was afraid of hurting other people's feelings if I spoke my anger. I was worried it would expose something about me others wouldn't like, which would disrupt my comfort and security. Instead, I used energy suppressing anger, either disguising it by saying I was upset or lying, saying there was no problem. I wanted to be the peacemaker, and I thought personal anger would only interfere. Not surprisingly, I often found myself in "un-selfed" positions in relationships.

My experience with Don gave me courage to deal with my own anger. I started telling myself, "It's okay to feel angry. Let it define your position and establish boundaries, Deborah. Expressing your anger is not necessarily going to make others stop loving you or cause them to reject you. Take a risk to be yourself."

I changed my language too. "I'm angry" was no longer foreign. Then I discovered an important secret about anger that totally changed my relationship with it. Each time I let myself feel anger, I could release it because it served its purpose of notifying me that I needed to either define myself in a problematic situation in which I had not been respected or I could decide to let the problem go if I determined my anger was unfounded.

I marveled at the vitality and genuineness I gradually gained as I let myself heal what I hadn't been letting myself feel.

Confronting Prejudice

Learning about veterans' stoicism and their various fighting-flighting-freezing-type behaviors was a slow and difficult process. It was also humbling. Somehow, early in my career, my idealistic mission to love veterans had yielded to criticism. Insidiously, a layer of cynicism and judgmentalism had attached itself to my arrogant and egotistical attitude about needing to "fix" veterans. My attitude silently distanced me from certain patients, particularly the younger ones, the ones about my own age who had served in Vietnam. I was put off by the long hair and tattoos so common among them, as well as the angry gruffness that seemed to go with the look. Sometimes they were jobless or homeless. In between hospital admissions, they seemed to spend their days drinking alcohol.

My ideal of "loving" evidently excluded these motley sorts though I'd never have admitted it. Certainly I provided the same care to them as anyone else, and I was always polite to them; but I maintained an emotional distance. Each time I had to admit another Vietnam veteran to the hospital with complications from alcohol abuse, I'd think, "Why can't they get their acts together?"

When I'd hear parts of their stories about their Vietnam experiences, I'd think scornfully, "Those are just excuses. The war's been over for years. They need to get over it and move on with their lives." I wasn't alone in my thoughts; other staff would join me in banter about Vietnam veterans' dysfuntionality. We knew they had been diagnosed with posttraumatic stress disorder (PTSD), but we trivialized their condition.

I also thought these vets had brought their troubles on themselves. They were often noncompliant. It was more evidence they purposely abused themselves and wasted my time. When I muttered a disgusted, "I don't understand these guys" statement to a colleague, I was more honest than I knew. I didn't understand, and I wasn't going to bother trying.

My time was in high demand. I walked fast and could dart up and down long hallways faster than a bullet from a high-powered military rifle. I was at my usual breakneck speed when I decided to pop in to a display of Florida veterans' artwork at the Medical Center. I had perfunctorily surveyed about half of the displays. Suddenly I was stopped in my tracks, struck by a painting of a soldier's face. I was surreally transfixed in time, unable to move. I was seeing what that soldier had seen, and it seemed like I was feeling what he felt. In his eye was a reflection of what he was seeing: suffering in the form of a burning hut. Though there were no people pictured, I knew they were inside the hut, dying. More importantly, the soldier's response portrayed tears of blood running down his face, signifying his loss of vitality. The painting was entitled, "Burning Vision." It was burning my vision too, igniting smoldering veteran prejudices, searing the filters from my eyes.

The same realness that had leapt off the canvas was evident in other paintings by the artist. Each gave me a perspective I had never experienced. Each drew me deeper into a world I didn't know. Each touched me in a place I wasn't sure I wanted to be touched, shedding light on those ugly places of dark, judgmental attitudes toward Vietnam vets. Frozen images of tattoos, long hair, alcohol abuse, divorce, joblessness, and homelessness melted before my eyes. "Why can't they get their acts together?" I'd always asked. Here was my answer. In that protracted moment where time and my deeper self stood still, the painting spoke.

I had a hard time going on with the rest of my day. I didn't know how to explain the change I had experienced. How do I describe going about my own business one minute and in an unguarded moment be healed of my prejudice? How do I explain that my carefully shielded-from-war world had just been shattered? How do I put into words how differently the world feels when arrogance and aloofness are replaced with understanding and connection?

The painting continued to haunt me. I decided to track down the artist, Tommy Bills.[2] Hesitantly I phoned him, telling him of my interest in his artwork. Tommy talked excitedly about his paintings and his healing. Finally (and reluctantly), I told him about the effect his painting had on my prejudice. Tommy assured me he was used to the prejudice expressed toward people with PTSD. He also described his many years of struggling with his addictions and dysfunctions while none of the numerous mental health care professionals he had seen ever delved into his history as a Vietnam veteran and its possible relationship to his problems. He himself had never brought it up because his disassociation with his painful past was so complete that he never correlated his bizarre behaviors to his Vietnam experiences. He began doing paintings and sculptures that seemingly had no connection to the war. Then a new psychologist saw the correlation and was able to help him begin dealing with it by painting about his experiences.

Tommy mailed me the diary that he had written as part of his recovery from PTSD. Now that my heart had been opened, I was ready to listen; I could bear witness to the suffering he had experienced.

I read it carefully. Like an old barnacled oyster shell pried open to reveal a luminous pearl, Tommy's diary exposed gems of understanding that lie beyond crusty, hardened surfaces. One entry read:

> A doctor told me to hold a compression bandage on the sucking chest wound of a young soldier who had a neat, round hole in the middle of his chest. He told me I was to keep my charge occupied "over there" because there were others who might still make it that he needed to work on. I kept assuring the sucking chest wound attached to the desperate soldier that we had the best medics anywhere.
>
> For just a moment, I let myself look beyond the gaping and the sucking. He had an all-American face and body. He had to have been my age, maybe even younger. No hair on his chest. Maybe he didn't even shave every day yet.
>
> The air gurgled in and out of his chest more loudly. With renewed determination, I increased my pressure on the bandage. If I pressed hard enough, surely I could make it stop. The gurgling became more muffled but no amount of pressure could muffle his pleas. He called out for his mother; he called out for God. Grabbing my arms, he

pleaded, "Please don't let me die"—not just once—
not just twice—but, over and over again. Each desperate plea increased my own desperation.

I remember the doctor telling me to "just
keep him quiet so he doesn't upset the others too
much." I don't know (and don't know if I want to
know) whether he died then or just passed out, but
they carried him away. Part of me wanted frantically to be carried away too.

There was still shooting around us. I remember crawling out of the building and seeing the
Sergeant-Major sitting on my jeep, just sitting out
in the open with all this firing going on. I made my
way to him to see if he knew the name of the guy I
had been caring for.

"Doesn't matter," he told me. "There'll be lots
more dying before this is over."[3]

Tommy's written words provided the context and meaning for
understanding his woundedness. I could now see the man behind the
soldier. I could see the vulnerable little boy hiding behind the hardened
wall. I now understood how the wall numbed and devitalized feelings.
I had seen that wall in hundreds of veterans. Now, I knew what was
behind it.

I realized other VA staff needed to understand the denial,
anger, pain, and acting-out behaviors generated by PTSD. So I
phoned Tommy to ask him about doing another art display at the
Medical Center for Veteran's Day. This display, however, would be
a one-man show. It would also give us an opportunity to meet face
to face.

When we saw each other, it seemed we had known each other
a lifetime. I laughed when I saw his ponytail. How differently I
experienced his façade now than I would have a few months earlier! I was also saddened. How many people had I failed to meet
because of the stranglehold of my biases? How many other stories

had I missed because they were hiding behind ponytails or tattoos or alcohol? How many healing opportunities had I missed because I didn't have the knowledge or courage to confront stoic walls of silence or anger?

Tommy joined my husband and me for dinner. It was fascinating to hear him speak with such vitality. The energy of his suppressed wounds was now released, enabling him to live authentically; he also no longer needed alcohol or drugs.

We were able to learn more about Tommy's "Burning Vision" painting that had made such a dramatic impact on me. He had painted it for a Marine veteran in his PTSD support group who had participated in unnecessarily burning down a village. "His guilt was so consuming that he was just a shell of man," Tommy told us. Tommy said the vet interacted well enough with the group, but whenever the topic of the burned village came up, he fell mute. Tommy had painted the picture to help the Marine express his feelings.

"Our whole nation needs healing," I had told Tommy and my husband when I heard this. "War is a loss of innocence for all of us, our whole country."

I thought about the loss of my own innocence during those years, telling Tommy how I had been a teenager and Vietnam didn't seem real; it was just a story on the nightly news. Then, one night I was struck by a news image showing soldiers carrying dead bodies out of a rice paddy. I turned the TV off and decided I wouldn't watch the news anymore.

My husband told Tommy about his pain when classmates never returned from Vietnam while everyone pretended life was unchanged. He talked about feeling guilty for not serving in the military himself. His father, a World War II veteran who annually attended First-Armored-Division reunions, had insisted his son remain in college to avoid the draft. The army had been important to his father. While other people bronzed baby shoes, his father's combat boots had been bronzed. They were footsteps memorialized on the living room mantle, but he had drawn the line when it came to risking his son witnessing what he had witnessed.

Listening to Tommy and my husband talking, I began to realize that war is the altar of sacrifice for a nation, an altar often unacknowledged by the civilian public. Soldiers have long had to shoulder the burden of adjusting to civilian life after they leave the military. It's often a long, lonely, and misunderstood journey to come back home. I saw that we needed to do more than just remember our veterans; we needed to re-member veterans into society.

The next day, Tommy and I did the presentation at the Medical Center.[4] Tommy explained how expressing his feelings through his artwork had helped heal the trauma he had experienced. I talked about my prejudices and how Tommy's paintings had helped me work through them.

I didn't anticipate the reaction of some of my colleagues. Just out of nursing school in the 60s, they had cared for the injured as the soldiers returned to the States a few days after receiving their war injuries. They, too, had blotted out their feelings. "I was just doing my job," most of them told me. They cried, however, as they said it, letting me see behind their wall. In those shared moments, we allowed ourselves to be the wounded healers that we are.

I also felt moved when two patients from the PTSD program made their way to my office the next day.

"You're the lady who spoke with the Vietnam vet yesterday aren't you?"

I nodded.

"We want you to have something." Each unpinned the yellow, green, and red-striped bar they had been given to indicate that he had served in Vietnam. "Thank you for giving us a voice. Thank you for wanting to understand."

"Oh no. I can't," I protested. "You don't understand. I've mocked and judged you all these years. I've done nothing to earn this honor."

"You're one of us now," they smiled forgivingly.

I knew how important these bars were to soldiers. Their willingness to relinquish something so precious emphasized how intensely they needed their voices to be heard and their suffering validated. Realizing resistance would ungraciously reject their generous gifts, I let them pin me with their symbol of sacrifice they were bestowing.

After they left, still stunned, I unpinned them, placing them on my desk. I was unworthy of their gifts. They were the heroes. I was but a witness, and I had been a reluctant one at that.

Growing Awareness Yields Lessons

- Stoic walls often "fight/flight/freeze" important emotions, emotions that generate vitality.
- It's okay to sensitively breach stoic façades, including my own.
- Healing begins when I let myself acknowledge my guilt, pain, anger, fear, and helplessness, and share it with others. "You can't heal what you don't feel."
- Instead of reinforcing stoic facades, look for opportunities to validate feelings.
- Make a decision to want to experience uncomfortable feelings and develop a strategy for doing so.
- Encourage deep breathing to create space for difficult feelings to be experienced.
- Anger holds an important secret. It notifies me that I need to either define myself in a problematic situation in which I have not been respected, or I can decide to let the problem go if I determine my anger is unfounded. Once I've done that, I no longer need the anger.
- The creative arts can be an important venue for healing trauma.
- Dare to go into ugly places of dark, prejudiced attitudes. It's amazing what can be discovered there.
- War is a loss of innocence for our whole country. We have to do more than just remember our veterans; we need to re-member veterans into society.

Chapter Three

Grin and Bear It

Stoicism is not strength to overcome,
but strength to hide.
Stoics develop an attitude of unshakability toward life,
a passionless calm
attained by an effort of strong will
and by a refusal to let one's self be touched
by the ordinary emotions of grief, hardship, and loss of life.
Stoics believe you should assert your mastery over outward events,
or, if you could not do that,
at least you should be unaffected by them."
—Rollo May[1]

In his diary, Tommy Bills had called the process of erecting his stoic wall "puttin' on the face." I wanted to know more about "the face" and how it gets "put on." I wanted to know how the military culture influenced these patients I was caring for. I wanted to better understand the relationship between their military history and their approach to health and illness. I realized, however, that I only cared for a small subset of veterans because only 15% of veterans receive care in the VA healthcare system. The average income of those receiving VA care is less than $10,000, with 25% reporting no income at all; 65% do not have a spouse.[2]

These veterans are similar and dissimilar from the veterans who do not receive health care in the VA. Like other veterans, they have served in different branches of the service; they held different ranks. Some had willingly enlisted; others had unwillingly enlisted; some had been drafted. Some had served in combat; others had not, though all had some combat training, and had to be willing to go to war if necessary. Some reported feeling lost after discharge from service, saying something to the effect of, "I left the shelter of my family for the shelter of the military. When I got out, I looked around and said, 'Now what?' I didn't know how to go on." Other veterans say just the opposite, reporting that the military provided direction and skills that helped them define themselves.

I listened carefully to their stories; they allowed me a privileged vantage point from which to discover a strange and unfamiliar world. They had joined the military for different reasons. Some joined to get away from situations. "I was just a pimply-faced, disobedient kid wanting to get away from home. I joined the military so I could get out on my own," one veteran told me. Others had gotten into trouble with the law and were told they could choose between the military or jail.

Many were motivated by patriotism. "I love this country. I couldn't think of a better way to serve than to become a soldier." Others joined for the benefits the military offered. They've told me things like, "I love to travel. I got to see the world." Some joined for the training and educational benefits that accompany service.

Some veterans had served unwillingly. One veteran said he didn't want to serve, "but I wasn't smart enough to go to college to maintain a deferment. I didn't want to move to Canada to avoid the draft. I had no choice." Some had served willingly, yet still suffered disappointment. One veteran told me he had signed up to go to Vietnam, but he was sent to join a unit in Europe instead. "I've always felt like I was only good enough to make the practice team; I could practice with the team, but I wasn't good enough to play." Some veterans have told me that they joined the military to avenge the death of a buddy killed in war.

Soldiers had a range of feelings about the training. Most told me that the military was the best thing that ever happened to them. Typically they would say something to the effect of, "It taught me how to grow up and become an adult." Others were ambivalent. They weren't necessarily glad or proud to have served. "I was forced to participate in something I didn't believe in," one veteran told me bitterly.

Basic training was grueling for some but the skills they learned were important because it would keep them alive in warfare. "Each of us was mentally torn down. It wasn't until we were completely broken down that we could be rebuilt," Joseph[3] told me. For others, it was demoralizing, as one veteran's perception reflects. "We were taught to shut up and listen. We were told that they didn't care about what we thought; the only thing they cared about was that we did what we were told. I came out feeling that I was insignificant and that no one cared." The tactics used to create a unified military team could be harsh. "When a recruit makes a mistake, he's singled out but everyone is disciplined for it. Individualism is poison when you're building a team-oriented fighting force. We succeed or fail together." They were taught control. "We were supposed to be perfectionists, down to the smallest detail—the way our shoes were shined and beds were made. The training helped us learn how to control our environment." Punishment was sometimes extreme. "Minor infractions might be met with having to clean floors and toilets with toothbrushes or exercising so vigorously we vomited."

The environment fostered camaraderie. "We would literally eat, sleep, shower, learn, laugh, cry, sweat, and bleed as a cohesive unit. All is shared and no one's ever left behind. We're taught to be our brother's keeper. The collective welfare always outweighs the needs of the individual." The risks of not being able to count on each other were high. "We were tested mentally and physically every day. It's important to find out who can adapt to difficult circumstances. Anyone who can't, poses a risk. We put our lives in the hands of our leaders and comrades each day. In this way, we gave each other life, or if mistakes were made, death."

Training got rougher when "kill-or-be-killed" instincts had to be developed. "We had to be able to kill automatically. Our lives and our comrade's lives depended on it. If you took time to think, you wouldn't pull the trigger and you'd get killed." Anger fuels instincts. "You can't kill someone you're not angry at." Training built endurance. "There are few greater sins in the eyes of a soldier than to fail or let other soldiers down. We'd rather die than fail or give up. We became more machines than humans." There were rites of passage that fostered strength. "When I was a new airman, the spiked metal wing pins were held against my chest while the other airmen pounded them until my undershirt was bloody."

Once training was completed, they sacrificed comfort. "Sometimes we lived in harsh living conditions. There were long deployments away from loved ones to hostile parts of the world. There was always the threat of death. And, sometimes, there was death itself." Physical scars were worn as a badge of honor. "They come with bragging rights. But emotional scars bring jeers. A soldier must be able to prove he has courage and can not only take pain, but have pride in the fact he can endure it so well. We can't show fear. Fear and pain are seen as signs of weakness. 'I can handle it' is our motto." They were taught how to live in survival mode. "In some ways, I've never come out of that mode. Some days I'm on automatic pilot—like a robot."

Some identify ambivalence with their role in society. "We bear the scars of our suffering as a badge of courage, yet we often suffer in silence. We pay the price demanded for the American way of life." Even after discharge, military service continued to exert its influence. "After I left, I lost my identity. I didn't fit in. I was straddling two worlds and didn't belong to either. I didn't even know how to settle a dispute or deal with conflicts that arose. All the rules had changed. Nothing was regulated anymore." They sometimes felt devalued. "I used to be important; other peoples' lives depended on me. Now, I'm a nobody." Some veterans have told me they had become "adrenalin junkies," causing them to drive recklessly or have difficulty adjusting to mundane civilian life. "I was used to action and drama. When I got home, I was bored. I wanted adventure."

One mother told me that her son had come home from Iraq feeling invincible. He was killed shortly after his return, riding his motorcycle recklessly.

Veterans also recognized the price their families paid. "I got the recognition, while my wife's sacrifices went unnoticed. She's the one who had to learn to maintain the house and car, balance the checkbook, give birth without me at her side, provide child care alone, console lonely children, take care of family emergencies, and attend funerals. She did this for months on end, without support, often with financial hardship, while constantly worrying I would be killed and not come home." Combat veterans have sometimes told me about the difficulty they have empathizing with other peoples' problems. They've seen the worst that humankind has to offer and everything else pales in comparison. "My girlfriend complained because she didn't have the right clothes to wear to a party. I got angry. I wanted to scream, 'I was a POW. . . . Let me tell you about things to complain about.' Instead, I walked out and never returned any of her phone calls."

Children paid a price too. One adult son of a career-military soldier identified himself as a "military brat." In a voice mixed with sorrow and anger, he asked me a series of questions: "Do you know how hard it was for a little boy to say good-bye to his Dad every time there was a skirmish in the world? Do you know what it's like to want to watch the news more than cartoons so you can find out whether your Dad is safe? Do you know how much damage was done to me every time my Dad left and the adults turned to me and said, 'You're the man of the house now'?" I could only nod numbly, but since that day, I've had a fervent hope that no adults will say those kinds of words to little boys or little girls.

The Marine Corps seems to be in a category all its own with especially effective indoctrinations. "Once a Marine, always a Marine" says the slogan. It's true. I can usually spot a Marine years after his military days are gone. They're tough; they face illness as though it were an enemy combatant. One Marine told me about a sign on their barracks: "Pain is weakness leaving the body." It explained why he didn't want to take pain medication for his advanced cancer he now had. Marines' deaths can sometimes be difficult. As one veteran told me, "You can't kill a Marine." It's true, they don't let go easily.

Though the Marine culture can sometimes complicate peaceful dying, there can be no doubt about its importance. The Marine culture brought thousands through harm's way safely. The instilled values were also often successfully applied to their civilian lives.

When I ask Marines how their beliefs became so ingrained, they tell me things like, "We were instilled with learning Marine Corps history, customs, and traditions that fostered a sense of pride and brotherhood. This was as important as the courses in survival, marksmanship, and hand-to-hand combat. It helped us feel an incredibly strong sense of belonging to something larger than ourselves. We drew on each other for strength. We could count on each other."

Then there's the Marine slogan of "the few, the proud." As one Marine told me, "It was instilled that we were special, better than any other platoon, better than any other branch of service, better than any other country. We were arrogant."

Sometimes it evidently went beyond arrogance. "We were taught that civilians don't care about us, are undisciplined, and have no regard for anything sacred in life other than their own self-gratification. This helped form our new identity, but it sometimes crippled us when we returned to civilian life."

For some, the military culture defined their existence: "We lived and still live by our Marine Corps motto: *Semper Fidelis* (a Latin phrase meaning "Always Faithful"). We are forever faithful to whatever God we choose to worship, our country, and our Corps. There's no room for those who would have it any other way. There are few 'gray areas' for us."

As I heard each veteran's story, I realized that as distinct as the military is from civilian society, it is also a reflection of it. The military gets the strong, the weak, the smart, the less-than-smart, the evil, the good, and the truly exceptional in the same proportion as the American citizenry. After induction, however, the creation of the rugged soldier who can "handle anything" started to emerge. Like a plant's spore whose hardened shell can endure the severest weather, germinating years later, military beliefs continued to exert their influence throughout their lifespan.

I began to realize part of the reason military indoctrination was so effective was because it occurred at an impressionable age when people were forming their young-adult identity. Away from family, with a desire to belong, young men and women defined themselves within the military culture, imprinting its belief systems. When recruits were issued a uniform, they clothed themselves in a new identity as well; remnants were often retained long after the uniform was gone.

I gradually developed an appreciation for the many difficulties soldiers returning to civilian life experienced.[4] They were used to being "out of country," and once discharged from active duty and assuming veteran status, they remained out of country even in their own country. While the rest of us had been spending our young adult years learning how to gain skills and knowledge to get along in the world, they were learning how to fight the world. Their relationships were often temporary, dissolving with the next set of transfer orders. Not only were the normal growth and developmental tasks of young adulthood bypassed, but they learned a culture that focused on protection and killing, which was sometimes at odds with day-to-day living. Often they didn't realize how much their experiences had changed them. "I thought I'd serve my country, come home, remove the uniform, and resume my life where I left off. I had no idea how life-changing those few years were. At that age, I was so naïve."

These indoctrinated beliefs did not always yield easily to new information or civilian culture. Even when military programs were offered that would help them adjust to civilian life, it was often refused because of their eagerness to return home. "I didn't want debriefing. All I wanted was to get back to my family. I'd been away long enough." Some cite naivety that often accompanies youthful thinking. "I thought I knew everything in order to go back to being a civilian. I didn't want to listen to others telling me what I thought I already knew." Soldiers seldom learned how to let go of stoic values that kept them from themselves and the ones who loved them.

It was my decision to confront stoicism that led to new discoveries. This decision didn't come easily or without serious discernment. I had been to conferences on grief and coping with cancer and death. I had consistently been taught to provide support for patients' own way of grieving, without trying to change them or impose my ways. In particular for people who were stoic, I had been taught I needed to respect their stoicism. Trying to coax them out from behind their wall of silence would be inappropriate. In theory I agreed with this. Yet, repeatedly, I had seen the damage stoicism could do to a patient when it was used as a means of negating the validity of their own experience.

Could there be a way to create a safe emotional environment where letting go of stoicism could be *offered* without being imposed? Perhaps we could think of the wall as a door instead, a door they could open or close at will and as often as they wanted, leaving the safety of their stoicism available to them. Maybe they'd be willing to come out once they'd experienced the vitality of the released energy they had disconnected from so many years before. Downplaying their suffering and ashamed of "weak" feelings, veterans often confused stoicism with courage. Maybe we could help them see another kind of courage—the courage to encounter uncomfortable emotions openly and without apology.

I decided to get better acquainted with the stoicism I encountered so frequently in veterans. I began with the dictionary.

"*Stoic:* showing indifference to joy, grief, pleasure, pain."[5]

I was staggered with the implications of the definition. In suppressing grief, stoicism also suppressed pleasure. Like spores that entomb potential energy and growth, stoicism walled off vitality, dividing inward and outward selves. Until the wall can be breached, vitality can not be accessed. I had seen this often, and families sometimes complained to me about their loved ones' remoteness from emotion.

It was then I realized that death was not the enemy. The enemies were those things that interfered with a *peaceful* death. Stoicism was at the top of that list, at least with many of the veterans I worked with. I decided then, I had to try to breach the wall. I would probably make some mistakes, and I might fail altogether; but I had seen stoicism rob too many people of a peaceful death. I had seen it keep people trapped in isolation, disconnected from those they loved and from their inner selves. Though I would continue to respect their silence when they chose to maintain it, I would also offer them alternatives.

One day, a doctor asked me to convince a patient named Steve to attend our emotional support group. "He's depressed," the doctor said. "The group will cheer him up."

Steve had malignant melanoma. His treatment had failed. Luckily for Steve, I'd grown beyond my earlier stage of trying to "cheer up" depressed patients. I entered the room ready to accept his feelings, willing to explore them with him. With downcast eyes and a flat voice, he told me how alone he felt.

"I'm a fighter and my family keeps telling me to keep it up," he said. "If I stop fighting, I'll be letting everyone down."

Recognizing the stoic wall for the isolation it was creating, I carefully and cautiously asked, "Are you ready to die, Steve?"

He shrugged his shoulders noncommittally.

"You need to know it's okay to die. If your time has come, then it's a matter of getting ready," I said gently. "Maybe you could tell your family that you're tired of fighting and that you need their help so you can die peacefully."

He looked in my eyes for the first time, moaning, "But I don't know how. I've never died before. I don't know how to do this."

Slowly I drew in close to him. "You didn't know how to be birthed into this world either, but your body knew how to bring you here. Your body has an inner wisdom. It knows how to take you back home. Trust it. Open up to it."

He nodded for an instant, then pulled back. "I can't," he said, shaking his head. "That would be giving up. I can never surrender."

"Surrender isn't good on a battlefield," I acknowledged. "But this isn't a battlefield, Steve. Dying is a natural part of life. It's a very important part of life."

Hesitantly, he nodded cautiously considering the possibility. We talked about the difficulty of preparing for death, the obstacles interfering with confronting it, and the advantages of both him and his family getting ready for it.

"Would it make it easier if I told them in your presence? Then you could talk about it together."

He smiled gratefully and told me he was expecting his daughter to arrive soon. When she did, I greeted her and let her know there was something important we needed to talk about. "As you've probably noticed, in spite of everything we're doing, your Dad's getting weaker. He's weary. He's ready to die, but he's afraid he's letting you down if he doesn't keep fighting."

As I spoke, his daughter started to cry. I paused, giving her time to absorb what I was saying, then I continued. "He's nearing the end of his life and he needs your permission to let go of the fight and open up to the reality of his approaching death. He's got a lot to face and he wants your help."

Several months pregnant, his daughter slowly turned to her father, kneeling down before him. "Daddy, I'm so sorry for telling you to keep fighting. I was being selfish because I didn't want you to go." Tearfully she explained why. "I just wanted my baby to know you. But now I realize that he *will* know you because I'll tell him about you. Your love for me will be the same love I give to him."

Steve reached out to her and they silently held each other. The daughter then hugged me, sobbing in my arms. "Thank you for caring enough to not let Daddy die alone," she whispered.

My talk with Steve gave me the confidence to approach others. I was lucky that he was the first, needing only a prod to help him let go and open up to the dying process. I knew others might not respond so easily. It had to be done carefully. I would have to go slowly, picking up on their cues. Each would have his own pace.

To gain veterans' trust, I had to become trustworthy. Confronting my own judgmental attitude had been the first step, an essential step. This step helped me become more authentic; authenticity is important. Veterans traumatized by war don't trust easily. They've been taught *not* to trust. Betray a combat veteran once, and you become the enemy. These veterans could sniff out a phony instantly, and they were quick to tell me there was nothing they disliked more. They were quite forbearing, however. If I said the wrong thing, if I took too long understanding what they needed, they for-gave easily; they understood human fallibility. What I couldn't do is pretend to understand what I didn't or fake confidence when I was uncertain. What I couldn't do was lie to them; this meant I couldn't lie to myself. Nor could I try to emotionally bully them into accept-ing my views. What I could do was en-courage them to face their hidden feelings and support their efforts to do so. By allowing myself to feel my feelings, I could help veterans feel their feelings. Some would choose to die as stoically as they had lived, and this too I needed to respect.

I discovered that inside most of my stoical patients was a gentle, sensitive human being just waiting for a chance to emerge. The vio-lent acts that many of these men committed didn't mean that they had no tenderness in them. Tenderness breeds compassion. It has to be covered up with a hardened shell in order to fight and kill. Unfortunately, the shell might remain when the war is over. Sometimes guilt or horror over what they have seen or done seals the shell, but this guilt often needs to be faced and felt so the soldiers can heal and come home to themselves.

Uncovering Tenderness: Pride and Prejudice Transformed

I wasn't the only one who helped our patients find and embrace their emotions. Others on the staff were learning the same skills I was. Sometimes transformation occurred among the patients themselves.

One of the most profound transformations I witnessed occurred between roommates who seemed like the odd couple. They had been strangers until fate found them in the same room on our Hospice and Palliative Care unit. Luke was a quiet, gentle man. He was par-alyzed by a spinal cord compression caused by prostate cancer. He was down to 100 pounds, and his body was contorted like a pretzel. He was also blind from glaucoma. Yet, he emanated serenity. He had a wonderful sense of humor and a youthful giggle that invited every-one into light-heartedness.

Luke also emanated gratitude. He was grateful to be alive, grateful to receive care, grateful even to be dying because he knew he would soon be home with "my Lord." As an elder in his church, Luke was well known and well loved in the town's African-American community. Now that he could no longer go to church, his family brought church to him: hymns, communion, scripture, and prayer. When none of his family was around, staff members would play recordings of the Bible or of Mahalia Jackson.

There was a genuine holiness in Luke; whenever he spoke, everyone in his presence felt this holiness. Everyone, that is, except his roommate.

Arthur was a gruff ex-Marine Corps sergeant. He admitted to being in pain, but usually refused medication. Instead, he paced. The effects of frostbite from inadequate footgear in the cold regions of Korea had caused some painful nerve damage to his feet; nevertheless, he was grateful that he hadn't had an amputation the way some of his comrades had.

As Luke had brought everyone into his serenity, Arthur brought everyone into his misery. He was a surly man with little tolerance for anyone's ways except his own. Divorced four times, he claimed all his wives had been stupid. He was estranged from his children, but his 41-year-old son, Frank, began to visit him. Not having seen his father for 30 years, Frank wanted one last chance to know him. Arthur frequently snarled and cursed at Frank. Yet, Frank remained undaunted and stayed faithfully at his father's side.

I made an effort to reach Arthur. "You seem so angry," I said. "It worries me to see how you're pushing everyone away from you."

He shrugged. "They're all morons, that's all," he said contemptuously.

"Is it possible," I asked lightly, "that *you're* the one being moronic at the moment?"

He scowled, but he didn't push me away.

"You really want everything to go your way," I continued. "Anyone who has other ideas is wrong."

"Yeah," he grunted. "You gotta problem with that?"

"That was important in the military. It worked well then. You were a sergeant and you needed your men to do what you told them to do, but I don't know about now. You might be facing the end of your life in the next several months," I said soberly. "Everything's changing. You might want to think about doing things a little differently now so you can get ready to have a peaceful death, a death *without* fighting."

Arthur didn't say anything, but I could see him mulling it over. "Maybe . . . " he said grudgingly and then quickly changed the topic. Motioning toward Luke's bed, he asked to have his room changed. When I asked why, he described a racial incident in the Marine Corps in which he had been reprimanded when a subordinate "played the race card against me." We talked about how this incident had intensified his racism. He said he had little use for a blind, paralyzed black man.

I had to resist the urge to move Arthur. It would easily resolve the problem, but it would avoid an opportunity for making needed inward changes.

"I'll ask Luke and see what *he* says," I replied. Arthur was used to calling the shots. I wanted him to know that Luke had a voice in this too. I didn't want Arthur's prejudice to affect Luke, but I also knew Luke could be a healing influence on Arthur.

I spoke with Luke. He was not fazed by Arthur's mean-spirited assaults. Used to bigotry all his life, Luke shrugged off Arthur's ill temper and laughed with understanding at the proposed room change. Though Arthur didn't like it, I decided not to move him to another room.

Over the ensuing weeks, Luke's aura of holiness slowly infiltrated Arthur's side of the room. Arthur complained less about having Luke as a roommate. Gradually, Arthur started seeking the peace he saw in Luke. In the middle of a lonely night, Arthur called to Luke. "You awake, Luke?"

"Yep."

"How about a prayer?"

Luke prayed, and Arthur seemed to surrender some of his anger and bitterness. The wall that had shielded his tender, vulnerable feelings was slowly crumbling. Arthur became more mellow with fewer outbursts of temper.

Luke and Arthur began sharing other things. When Luke's family brought communion, Arthur had communion too. When Arthur went home on the weekends, he would bring back food to share with Luke. Frank talked to the staff to get approval to use the stove in the kitchen on the unit so he could make breakfast for his father; Arthur asked him to make enough for Luke too. When Frank fixed breakfast the next week, Arthur invited the other eight patients on the unit. Mahalia Jackson and the smell of bacon called everyone within hearing and smelling distance into satisfying repast. Soon the weekly event outgrew Frank's capabilities; volunteers and the hospice chaplain and physician were recruited into cooking, singing, and praying. Word of good food and fellowship spread throughout the Medical Center. Each week new faces from other wards eagerly appeared. (A tradition was born 12 years ago that continues to thrive today and has had the surprising effect of providing "pre-hospice" care for non-hospice patients.)

The friendship between Luke and Arthur deepened over their weeks together. Possibly for the first time, Arthur was caring about someone other than himself. When Luke needed something, Arthur was there to get it. Conversation drifted between their beds at all hours. A synchrony emerged as though they were still soldiers bonded in the same trench.

One morning as the sun was rising, Luke called out, "You awake, Art?"

"Yeah. What do you need Luke?"

When Luke didn't respond, Arthur sat up so he could see him more clearly. Luke lay there with his hand outstretched toward Arthur. "I'm dying, Art. The Lord is here for me."

"I'll get someone," Arthur said in a panic. Hurrying from the room, he returned with the housekeeper, Margurite. Luke smiled as the three joined hands. Arthur asked Margurite to pray. When they opened their eyes after the prayer, Luke had died.

Arthur was heart-broken. He beckoned to me as I came down

the hallway.

"Luke died, Deborah. I can't believe it. He died." He told and retold their last moments together as if to convince himself of the reality. I put my hand on Arthur's shoulder and said nothing. After awhile, he spoke again but he wasn't speaking to me or to anyone in particular. "Tell Luke I'll be joining him soon."

Arthur was given time alone with Luke, but at last it was time to prepare Luke's body for the morgue. Arthur's fierce Marine loyalty would not allow him to leave the room.

"I'm staying right here with him. I'm not going to abandon him now." The room was a foxhole from which these two had faced death together. Luke had carried Arthur through its fire. Now, it was Arthur's turn.

Arthur lingered at the doorway, watching as Luke's body was placed on a morgue cart. As Luke's body passed, Arthur raised his hand into a stiff salute. "There goes my best friend," he said, tears streaming down his face as the cart clattered down the hall. "Who would have ever thought . . . ," he added, his voice trailing off.

I could only remain silent, tears in my eyes, beholding the moment. I was filled with admiration for Arthur's courage and humility. I felt awed by the crumbling walls of prejudice Luke had penetrated. I had witnessed this kind of heroism in many veterans, but still I remained filled with wonder.

Arthur was now inconsolable. "How could Luke leave me?" he moaned despairingly.

Over the next few days, Arthur erected his wall again, becoming gruff and demanding. Nothing satisfied him, including his new roommate. No matter what his roommate said or did, it was wrong; it was not Luke. The roommate was moved and the bed kept empty for awhile to help Arthur focus on his grief. The empty bed seemed to contain Luke's spirit so that the Arthur that Luke had so lovingly coaxed from hiding, gradually reemerged.

Arthur's condition stabilized, and he was discharged to the Medical Center's community living center. Each week he reappeared for breakfast on the Hospice and Palliative Care Unit, usually with a few new buddies. Making new friends was no longer difficult; caring for other people was no longer foreign. Black or white, rich or poor, Arthur befriended everyone around him. His relationship with Frank grew tender; he had become the father Frank always wanted.

A year later, Arthur was readmitted to the Hospice and Palliative Care unit for end-of-life care. With Frank at his side, he died peacefully. It had been a year of change, a year with kinship and camaraderie. He had discovered the meaning of fatherhood and life without the specter of bigotry foreshadowing his perceptions. It had been a year of healing.

His memorial service was an apt metaphor for Arthur's transformation. Frank requested that the Hospice and Palliative Care team perform the service under a tree where Arthur and his friends had often gone to smoke during that last year. We could only imagine the amusement on Arthur and Luke's beatific faces as they heard their story recounted and watched us dance to Mahalia's booming voice. No doubt, Arthur and Luke were dancing with us. As Arthur, himself, had said, "Who would have ever thought . . . "

Though veterans like Arthur helped me understand the need to penetrate stoicism, I sometimes had to remind myself that there were important reasons it had been needed. Stoicism is necessary on the battlefield, as it is in many life situations; but the walls that stoicism erects soon outlast their usefulness. The walls keep out necessary feelings—and other people. Stoic "indifference" can be experienced by others as cold, uncaring detachment. Rigid control can be necessary in military environments but it backfires when it's used with loved ones.

Stoicism can create protection from untrustworthy influence in anyone's life for a time; but as a long-term coping mechanism, it can be stifling. It's the *relationship* to stoicism that needs modification. Its overuse creates problems as serious as the problems it has been used to counteract.

Over the years I've worked with veterans, I've seen that stoicism is made up of three components: pride, control, and independence. Some loved ones might even describe this determined pride as "stubborn." Control might be so intense that others describe it as "domi-nating." Independence is frequently cited as "fierce." Anything threatening pride, control, or independence can incite anger and defensive fight/flight responses.

Dying is a humbling experience that challenges all of these. You lose much of your control, your pride takes a blow, and your inde-pendence is taken away. Sooner or later, the wall has to crumble. Later means fighting to the bitter end; sooner means a weary soldier is final-ly able to surrender to hope for a peaceful death. It means scattered pieces of inward self are finally able to make peace with each other.

If unable to let go of pride, control, and independence so a patient can reach out for help, suffering might even be increased. However, letting go of these qualities takes work just as creating them does. Physical limitations and emotional displays can embar-rass the patient and create fears that others will perceive him as weak. It can make him feel helpless and vulnerable to attack. Veterans sometime view letting go as admitting defeat or an act of surrender, something good soldiers don't do. They might need support in re-framing these beliefs.

Mature mental health includes identifying our needs and asking for help when it is needed. Both require vulnerability. Stoicism often keeps people from saying what they need or allowing others to meet their needs. This mask of invulnerability sometimes won't even allow them to admit they *have* needs. This attitude can cause frustration, not only for themselves but for their families or professional care-givers. Fear of vulnerability can also prevent veterans from seeking or accepting help for depression or PTSD.

Pride can foster arrogant "I'm right and no one can tell me I'm not" stances. Inability to say "I'm sorry" or "I was wrong" interfere with reconciliation efforts. Pride can prevent people from acknowl-edging failing health, weakness, or other changes. It might mean not listening to one's own body or working beyond the point that the body is saying it is tired. Pride keeps people from seeking medical help, ignoring or belittling symptoms until it is too late to do any good. It can even keep people from admitting that they are dying. I try to help them let go of pride so new worlds can open.

Control increases the chance of conquering enemies on a battle-field; being vulnerable can get you killed. However, trying to control people or circumstances off the battlefield sometimes *creates* enemies. Fear of being at the mercy of others causes resistance. Family members sometimes speak about how simple conversations about relationship problems make the veteran feel like he's being controlled. When the need to control manifests as a need to conquer, it can create frustration, anger, and bitterness for everyone involved.

There is nothing like death to make us realize how little control we have. Yet, once made to realize that they are going to die, veterans sometime want to control its timing, getting angry and frustrated with the waiting. "I'm not dead and I'm not alive. If things can't go back to how they used to be, then let's get this over with *now*." Sometimes they even think they can control death itself. One patient told our team that we shouldn't be telling patients that it's okay to die. "You should be telling them to get more courage so they can get up out of these beds and fight death." Then he looked at me. "And you. You're the Director of this Hospice. If you had that as your mission statement, I bet you'd be on the cutting edge of hospice because no one else would be doing that." Our team had to suppress our desire to giggle because the patient was quite serious. Defend and control instincts are difficult to let go of. This man had no way of knowing that peace awaits those who are able to do so.

Fierce independence seldom yields without a fight. "I can handle it myself" is simply not always true. Nothing is more embarrassing than for a proud and independent veteran to have to ask for help with personal needs. Yet at some point, weakness forces realization of the necessity of dependence on others, unless you're a stoic veteran. Veterans have been taught to survive; they've received wilderness training. They pull themselves up by their own bootstraps. The imposaphobiacs that they are, they don't need help from anyone. This attitude causes frustration for family members who desperately want to do whatever they can. Independence often requires strong will power; ultimately, will power must also be surrendered.

Daily I see many of these veterans let go of control, allowing themselves to become completely human, growing in humility as they learn how to ask for help and how to become a gracious receiver, discovering connection and compassion in the process. This takes courage, and it is as heroic as facing any enemy in battle.

I've come to realize it is my admiration of veterans' humility, courage, and honesty to deal with the effects of stoicism and/or war trauma that makes working with them such a privilege. They reveal wisdom I need for my own life, and it starts with confronting my own prideful ways in which I have a hard time saying "I don't know," "I'm sorry" or "I was wrong." I'm confronted with my own controlling ways in which I think I'm God, not accepting my humanity with its risks and limitations. I'm confronted with my stubborn independence and the difficulty I have in identifying my needs or asking for help.

I've discovered that courage is not about covering up and "putting on a good face" nor is it about "being strong" by hiding behind stoic walls. I've discovered that not only is there no shame in being human, but also there is freedom in being able to acknowledge it and fully experience it. This is not a weakness; rather it requires strength and courage.

I've often identified myself as a "recovering coward." I attribute the recovering to the infusions of courage I receive each day as I witness veterans facing their deaths while learning how to set aside bricks from their stoic walls, one by one. It's not an easy process. "The hardest journey to make is the 12-inch journey from the head to the heart," is a hospice adage that I witness every day with stoic veterans; but it's also true for many others. American culture with its heritage of "rugged individualism" reinforces stoic values. Religions sometimes equate stoicism to faith. I was counseling a grief-stricken veteran whose son had committed suicide just a few weeks earlier. He told me that his pastor had told him that he was to bear his grief in private. He was told that it was his opportunity to "show others how strong your faith is." I shudder to think about the damage this kind of misguided advice causes.

The 12-inch journey from the heart to the head is no less difficult and no less important either. I was providing bereavement counseling with Judy, a woman whose husband had died. She had no
trouble feeling her grief. She had asked to see me because she could-
n't contain it. "I go to work and all I do is cry," she told me. "I'm
reduced to a puddle that won't dry up even after all these months. If
I don't get this under control, I'm going to lose my job."

"There are some things you can do to regain control," I told her.
I explained that she could make the trip from her heart to her head
by making a decision to "dry up the puddle" at work and "repuddle"
when and where she wanted. Ultimately, Judy decided my office was
the best place for "puddling." I told her that when she was at work
and her heart moved up to become a lump in her throat, her head
was to tell it, "Go back down. You can come out when I get to
Deborah's office in a few days."

When Judy crossed my threshold the next week, she burst into
tears for about two minutes, followed by an outburst of laughter. "I
can't believe it. I did it!" She discovered the value and power of exerting her "head" to provide needed safety and control.

Developing stoicism was important for Judy. It is valuable for all
of us when protection is needed or unsafe environments threaten
emotional harm. Stoicism can help prevent us from getting lost in
emotions. I sometimes light-heartedly say to overly-emotional or
underly-thinking patients, "Time to get a backbone" or "Get a grip"
or "Fake it 'til you make it." These are all ways of saying, "A little stoicism might help."

My concern about stoicism is when it is used inappropriately to
block energy and emotion from self or how stoicism interferes with
expressing love to others. My concern also stems from seeing how
"positive thinking" is sometimes used as a stoic front for denying
"negative" feelings. Unfortunately, the energy of those feelings has no
place to go except into unconsciousness. Paradoxically, the feelings
they most fear and want to avoid ends up controlling them. Positive
thinking is important but not when it's misapplied to hide us from
ourselves by denying the authenticity of our feelings. As one veteran

told me, "Every time I hide behind a stoic wall, I devalue myself. I'm valuing other people's opinion more than honoring who I am."

After suffering is validated and feelings acknowledged and felt, it is often most helpful to use stoicism as a means of navigating the world. I've written about the negative effects of stoicism because veterans often use it extensively as a habitual way of Fighting/"Flighting" others and self. My hope is that control over putting up and letting down a stoic wall is increased.[6]

Insight Revealed

My hope for all our veterans and their families is that we can help them gain a deeper sense of their lives, as well as a deeper sense of ourselves, so we can find peace together. To do that, we have to realize that there are aspects of veterans that may be different from their civilian counterparts.

I've thought a lot about what makes some of our veterans "tough, crusty characters," as VA staff often affectionately and sometimes not-so-affectionately call them. Initially, I wasn't able to specifically identify the common elements that contribute to the hardened VA culture. I wasn't able to articulate why taking care of tough veterans was different from civilians or why their deaths sometimes seemed complicated by their military experience. After more than 25 years caring for them, I now can. The conclusions I've drawn are:

- The value of stoicism so earnestly and necessarily indoctrinated in young soldiers might interfere with peaceful deaths for all veterans, depending on the degree to which stoicism permeated their later lives;
- Combat veterans' deaths might be further complicated by traumatic memories or paralyzing guilt, depending on the extent to which they were able to integrate and heal traumatic or guilt-inducing memories;
- A high incidence of alcohol abuse[7] or other "flighting"-type behaviors are often used either to avoid confronting locked-up

feelings or to numb traumatic memories;
- Veterans often acquire wisdom from having reckoned with trauma, stoicism, and addictions.

For us to access this last element, it's helpful to understand the previous three.

Lessons Learned about Military Culture

- The military is a reflection of people in society. After induction, however, the stoic soldier who can "handle anything" is commonly created.
- I have concluded that stoicism is made up of three components: pride, control, and independence. Anything threatening pride, control, or independence can incite anger and defensive fight/flight responses.
- The value of stoicism so earnestly and necessarily indoctrinated in young soldiers might interfere with peaceful deaths for all veterans, depending on the degree to which stoicism permeated their later lives.
- Veterans often downplay their suffering and are ashamed of "weak" feelings.
- Inside most stoical patients is a gentle, sensitive human being just waiting for a chance to emerge. Tenderness is covered up with a hardened shell in order to fight and kill.
- Stoicism is important, even essential, especially on a battlefield. It creates protection from untrustworthy influences. It's the *relationship* to stoicism that needs modification. Its overuse creates problems as serious as the problems it has been used to counteract. It can be used inappropriately to block energy and emotion from self or interfere with expressing love to others.
- Combat veterans' deaths might be further complicated by traumatic memories or paralyzing guilt, depending on the extent to which they were able to integrate and heal traumatic or guilt-inducing memories.
- Veterans traumatized by war don't trust easily. To gain their

trust, I have to not only confront my own judgmental attitude, but also allow myself to feel my feelings. This attitude can help veterans feel their feelings.

- A high incidence of alcohol abuse or other "flighting"-type behaviors are used either to avoid confronting locked-up feelings or to numb traumatic memories.
- Courage is not about covering up and "putting on a good face" nor is it about "being strong" by hiding behind stoic walls. Not only is there no shame in being human, but there is freedom in being able to acknowledge and fully experience it. This is not a weakness; rather it requires strength and courage.
- Veterans often acquire wisdom produced from having reckoned with trauma, stoicism, and addictions.
- There is much that we can do to create safe emotional environments for veterans (See Appendix B).

Chapter Four

Wounds of War

Does your spirit know
that by my killing you
I also killed
a part of myself?
—*Looming* by Karl Michaud[1]

I've taken care of many veterans who have been in war. Some have not only been in one war, but two; some have even been in three. I have never seen *any* war, but I have witnessed its effects.

It wasn't until I had worked for many years in the VA system and heard many stories from veterans that I realized the impact these effects had. Many effects were good. Though a few soldiers were motivated for self-glorification and promotion, most were motivated for different reasons. They didn't fight for themselves; they were mostly selflessly motivated to fight for a cause and to fight for comrades. They were willing to lay down their lives for each other; many exhibited extraordinary acts of bravery to preserve their buddies' survival or accomplish an important mission. Many effects were not good. I've come to realize how people who sustain trauma sometime sustain emotional, mental, social, spiritual, and moral injuries that can cause a lifetime of suffering.

Another important lesson my patients taught me was that each war was different. Each had its own culture that exerted a different influence on young soldiers. World War II was enthusiastically supported by Americans. Many veterans have told me they joined when they were 16, lying about their ages so they could fight. When one veteran told me he had been 14, I could only shake my head in wonderment.

Virtually everyone sought a way to support World War II. People grew "victory gardens" and the Red Cross sent pictures of them to the soldiers so they could see their country's support. Women worked in munitions factories while others stayed home and made clothing for the soldiers. No one was left untouched.

Without televisions, the public could be shielded from war's brutality. War could be glamorized, which increased its appeal and fostered national unity. The mission of World War II enhanced this unity; it was clear and largely undisputed—especially after Pearl Harbor. The soldiers knew they were in the war for its duration. This fostered cohesion and a determination to get the mission accomplished—a "we're in this together until the job gets done" attitude. When the war was over, troops came home together. They were greeted as heroes by a public eager to hear their victorious wartime stories.

While the adulation was gratifying, the soldiers needed more from their friends, families, and the media. They had been through horrors they could not have imagined; they had done things they never thought they would do. They needed the approval they were getting, but they also needed to give voice to the traumas they had suffered. The awaiting public, however, only wanted to hear about acts of bravery and heroism, not of trauma and moral confusion. The soldiers themselves often downplayed their acts of courage. "The real heroes were those that didn't come home" or "I was just doing my duty." This kind of reticence was sometimes taken for modesty, but some have told me that it's not modesty. They don't feel like heroes because they knew the ugly, despairing, or cowardly acts of war. "If you knew what I did, you wouldn't think I was so heroic." These stories often remained untold, lurking in the veterans' consciousness, hiding guilt and shame.

The Korean War was different. My Korean War veterans are often more tight-lipped. Known later as the "Forgotten War," it was never an officially declared war; rather, it was called a "Conflict" or "Police Action." There were no ticker tape parades for these returning soldiers. This time was the happy 1950s and people wanted to forget about war and focus on growing prosperity. Korean soldiers' trauma had been minimized or neglected and their combat contributions sometimes forgotten.

If Korea taught us how to ignore soldiers, Vietnam taught us how to shame and dishonor them. There was extensive television coverage from Vietnam. Americans now understood the brutality of war, and many were at odds with its politics. Protests were organized across college campuses. Actress, Jane Fonda, sent much-publicized cookies to the enemy, an act that symbolized a divided nation.

Many young men had mixed feelings about the Vietnam War, and some opposed it. The draft forced these and others into military service and then into combat. Also, imposed beliefs from fathers who were World War II veterans sometimes prompted unwilling sons to volunteer for Vietnam. For others, sons sought the hero status their World War II fathers had held in the family (and usually came back disappointed, I notice).

These soldiers often became more cynical by their experience in Vietnam, and their cynicism affected the soldiers who believed the war was necessary. This prevailing mood is depicted by a caption on a painting in the National Vietnam Veterans Art Museum in Chicago. It reflects the bitterness I often saw corroding the souls of some veterans. It read:

> We the willing
> Led by the unknowing
> Do the necessary
> For the ungrateful[2]

In addition to political influences, there were pragmatic factors. Though they could volunteer for more, soldiers were required to do only one-year tours in Vietnam. Rather than the attitude of "we're in this together until we get the job done" of World War II soldiers, they tended to think in terms of "I'm just rotating through until my tour's up." Reports of antiwar protests at home shook their confidence in the war as well.

Frequently-rotated new troops also meant fewer available seasoned troops. "You couldn't trust new soldiers to cover your back," a Vietnam vet told me. He said green recruits were also more trigger happy. "They were more likely to kill our own soldiers who they mistook as enemy soldiers."

War tactics also were different in different wars. Before Vietnam, there was a certain level of safety "behind the lines" (if there can be any safety in a war), which allowed a small degree of mental and emotional recuperation between battles. In Vietnam, however, it was guerilla warfare; there was no safe place to let defenses down. The enemy easily infiltrated, making it difficult for soldiers to distinguish friend from foe. Soldiers were on guard even in their sleep. Explosives were sometimes hidden on dead bodies, blowing up when soldiers came to retrieve them. Commonly, I've heard stories of soldiers carrying food on them so they could give it to village children; but this could be used against them. Sometimes, the children were booby-trapped to explode while in the soldiers' midst!

As important as any of the military factors was how the non-military public treated Vietnam veterans. Unlike World War II veterans, these men and women were not welcomed as heroes. Often they weren't welcomed home at all. Antiwar protests had grown and people who had advocated bringing the soldiers home now turned their anger against the soldiers themselves. They greeted returning soldiers at the airports by spitting on them and shouting "baby killers" or "murderers." As a result, soldiers often hid their history about Vietnam like a dirty secret.

I've often speculated about how differently our soldiers would have been treated had there been a convincing victory in Vietnam. The reality is, however, that Americans don't like losers, even in war, even when it may not have had anything to do with the warriors. We didn't want to hear; we wanted no reminders. As a result, soldiers' stories had nowhere to go. They couldn't even talk with each other much of the time. Unlike World War II soldiers who often came home in boats or trains that gave them time to share their experiences and "debrief" each other along the way, Vietnam soldiers were flown home into a hostile civilian culture in a single day. Their suffering was never validated, their souls left burdened, their stories left untold because we didn't want to hear them.

I've often watched World War II veterans rightfully swell up with pride when Hitler is mentioned. "We got him," they'll say feeling the satisfaction of being part of a successful campaign to protect the world from evil. Vietnam veterans rarely feel this kind of satisfaction. Uncertainty and ambiguity about the goals and outcomes of the war often erode any sense of achieved purpose. Without a convincing victory, veterans felt their sacrifices had been meaningless. The political nature of the war added to their sense of injustice. "We could have won that war if the politicians had stayed out of it," some vets have told me. "They never financed the war so that we could have the resources to do what needed to be done," others have said. "They sent us in there knowing we couldn't win." This sense that their sufferings had been futile could linger for years, corrupting their civilian lives and even their deaths years later.

When I started seeing how isolated Vietnam veterans were, I often encouraged them to join the Veterans of Foreign Wars, American Legion, or Disabled American Veterans organizations. "We're not welcome there," I was told sometimes. "They don't understand us either." Some World War II vets couldn't comprehend that Vietnam was different. Some viewed these soldiers as "wimps" who had "lost" the war. I remembered all the quips TV's Archie Bunker made about the superiority of World War II: "the *big* one" (i.e., the *only* one). The generational clash and the war culture clash interfered with communication and support. Initially, the Veterans of Foreign Wars posts did not allow Korean or Vietnam vets to join because those wars were not declared wars. Though that is no longer the case, it has taken years for the American public to register more understanding and acceptance; for most Vietnam vets, the damage had already been done.[3]

Postcombat Trajectories

I didn't always realize that soldiers never escaped war unscathed. I didn't realize it because I didn't ask questions about their combat experiences; or I didn't know how to ask the questions in a manner that yielded meaningful answers; or I didn't know how to penetrate stoic walls; or I didn't have a trusting relationship with veterans so they could be forthcoming; or I wasn't trustworthy enough because I was still a phony; or I didn't really want to hear about combat recovery or hadn't realized its relevance to their dying. Once I learned how to penetrate walls and once I realized the relevance of combat history, I started paying attention to the relationship between combat history, postcombat integration of trauma (or its lack), and the quality of death (turmoil vs. serenity).

I have nursed more than five thousand veterans as they've faced dying; a large percentage of these men and women have been combat veterans. As I've listened to the effects of war on their lives, I notice some combat veterans have an easy time approaching the ends of their lives; others have a more difficult time. I've often speculated about rationales for the varying responses. In an overly simplified and generalized way, my speculations have led me to conceptualize war as a black hole with no light of day, no consciousness. Like black holes in the universe that suck life from surrounding space, war sometimes sucks the life out of soldiers. When they return home from war, they want to just leave the war behind them and get on with their plans for their future. Their ability to do this varies; I conceptualize this variance along a spectrum of three trajectories:

- True integration and healing of postwar trauma
- Apparent integration of combat trauma with the veteran seemingly unscathed until combat memories escape from behind stoic walls as they face personal illness, death, or some other trigger
- Incomplete integration of trauma (PTSD)

I've also wondered if a determining factor of which trajectory is taken might depend on the strength of a veteran's stoic wall to encapsulate, segregate, and isolate them from healing resources within the self. Those on trajectory 1, for example, might somehow fail to build a stoic wall or they might remodel it in such a way that it does not isolate them from themselves or others. People on trajectory 3, on

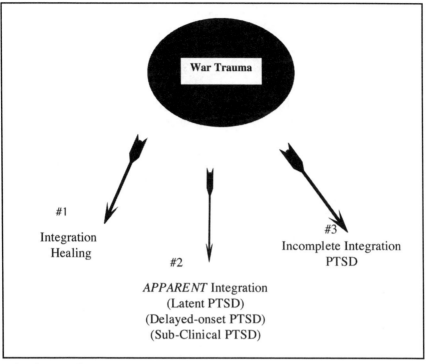

This diagram shows possible outcomes following trauma.

the other hand, might build walls that end up imprisoning them-selves because it takes a lot of energy to deaden experiences that are alive with emotion.

I've thought a lot about the people on trajectory 2. One thought I have had is that they may have erected a wall without realizing it. This unknown barrier is lost in a consciousness that can't see it, feel it, or find its way through it.

Trajectory 1: Integration of Trauma

I've worked with veterans of all categories as they come to the ends of their lives. My observations have led me to speculate that to the extent to which people reckon with trauma *before* they come to the end of life, is the extent to which they will have a peaceful death. In general, combat veterans of the first category who have struggled and successfully reckoned with their combat experiences, have a better end-of-life experience than the rest of us are going to have. They've had to go into a deeper part of themselves to reconcile the horrors they have faced, including confronting their own mortality at an early age; most of us have been spared this unsettling task.

"I've faced death before in the war. I'm not afraid of it anymore." I hear this often from veterans on trajectory 1, those who've successfully integrated war trauma into their lives. They say it sincerely without stoic "macho" bluster. They say other things too:

"Every day since the war has been a gift, each day a day I didn't think I'd have."

"But for the grace of God, it could have been me who died in that war. I'm aware of the gift of grace with me now as I'm facing death."

"I must have been spared in that war for a reason. I've lived my life trying to live up to the reason, to fulfill that meaning. If I don't do that, it means my buddies died for nothing."

For them, war did not erect a stoic wall. It tore one down. War brought focus and changed priorities. "It made me see what was *really* important." All else pales after having experienced the worst humankind has to offer. Perspectives shift, and often shift toward a willingness to reckon with any obstacle interfering with peace, including inward obstacles. They often have a resiliency that transcends victimization. Rather than identify with their trauma, they identify with the lessons they learned from war and its recovery. Rather than perpetuating violence, they perpetuate peace.

While the rest of us so often delude ourselves into thinking we're immune from death, these veterans on trajectory 1 realize death is always at their sides. In the process, they seek reconciliation in their relationships, express love, and demonstrate gratitude. Death adds richness to their lives, helping them live beyond their egotistical or material selves. Paradoxically, death helps them tap into unconscious energy, awakening a passion for life. They have lived their lives better because of their war experience.[4] The cruelty of war taught them how to love and forgive others and themselves. It was a lesson they lived daily. Because they faced death before and lived their lives differently, they live their deaths differently, but it requires hard work like this next veteran's story demonstrates.

Heroic Journeys after War

Milton was frail and wilted, a blanket drawn tightly around his shoulders as he sat staring out the window. I was answering a hospice consult from his physician to see if he was appropriate for care on our Hospice and Palliative Care unit. My mission was to gain a sense of this 82-year-old man's story and what had been important to him, his current struggles as he reckoned with deteriorating health, and his hopes for his coming death.

"Everything is wonderful because I have a room with a beautiful view," he said when I asked about how he was doing.

I wasn't sure how to respond. So often the phrase, "everything is wonderful," is used stoically to avoid reckoning with a grim personal world. In those situations, the last thing I want to do is reinforce the denial. I didn't know this man yet or what his "wonderful" meant. There was a quiet vitality about him that made me trust his sincerity; I had no sense of stoic false bravados.

I noticed a notebook of stunning watercolor paintings by his bedside; some were recent sketches of the view from his window in the hospital.

"Did you do these?" I asked, impressed.

"Oh, yes," he responded with enthusiasm.

"How did you come to develop such an appreciation for nature and beauty?" I said as I leafed through his notebook of sketches.

"Oh," he chuckled, "It's easy. That's an artist's job." He began to talk about his local fame as an artist commissioned by the city, as well as the paintings he did during his travels to India. He saw my interest in the latter, and pulled out a portfolio of watercolors when he lived there.

I told him of my own travel to India, the hospice I had visited

there, and how I, too, had stayed in the homes of locals. "Your paintings bring me back," I told him. "I found India to be a fascinating
land of incongruities," I told him.

We were both delighted to discover a fellow pilgrim who had
experienced the enigmas of India. We reminisced about our similar
adventures in a land so different from our own. I talked about how
the trip had been a turning point in my life; it had forced me to let
go of my fear of the unknown and open up to uncertainty and ambiguity.

As much as I wished to continue our talk about India, I needed
to return to the task at hand. "From the outside, you sound like
everything's going well. I'm wondering how things are going on the
inside?"

"Ah, on the inside? . . . is bliss." He said it with strength, joy,
and clarity, drawing me into rapt attention.

"But everything's falling apart," I protested. "You're getting frail.
Each day is becoming a struggle. You might be nearing the end of
your life."

"I have bliss because God is with me no matter what. It doesn't
matter what is happening with my body. It doesn't matter what is
happening out there. In here," pointing to his head and then his
heart, "is bliss. It doesn't change."

"Is that because of your religion?" I asked.

"My *religions*," he corrected me smiling. "I believe in all religions. They lead to the same place—to a place of bliss. I've learned
to practice them all," he said with serenity and security.

"I'm wondering how you came to live this wisdom," I said
intrigued. "I know it wasn't just by reading books or living in India
or practicing all religions or being an artist. It had to be born from
something beyond that, struggles transcended no doubt. What did
you do in the military? You haven't mentioned that part of your life
yet." If he was being stoical, this is where it would come out.

He became still, pensive. "Well, yes. That would be it . . . " He
said no more.

"That would be what? I don't understand," I asked after a few moments.

"I was a POW you know," he said, turning to look me fully in the eyes. "I was tortured in a German war camp."

There was no self-pity in his voice. I could see he was at peace with his memories so I didn't press for details. "War brings out the worst in people," Milton said. "But it also brings out the best." He then told me how he was watching a documentary on TV about an American POW who had been imprisoned next to a cell with Russian prisoners. The walls between them didn't extend completely to the ceiling. The Russian prisoners overheard how the American prisoners were starving to death. "Do you know what the Russian prisoners did?" Milton asked me.

I shook my head.

"They threw pieces of bread over the wall to the Americans. When I heard that on the TV, I started sobbing. I couldn't stop." He paused to see if I grasped the significance of what he was saying. He clarified. "They were starving too. Not only that. Do you know what would have happened to them if they would have been caught?"

"I would guess they would have been shot," I conjectured.

Milton nodded. We sat quietly together while I marveled at what he had seen and experienced. Then I asked him how he was able to reckon with his experiences in the POW camp. "If those things had happened to me, I'd be bitter," I added.

"I was at first," he said. "After I was released, I wanted nothing to do with Germany or with Germans. I cringed just to hear a German word; it brought back memories of guards spitting out German words as they tortured us. I had moved on in my life. I was an art professor at the University of Southern California. I didn't need to remember."

Events in his life forced him to remember, however. The phone rang one day and he heard a woman with a German accent. It was Friendlinde Wagner, Richard Wagner's granddaughter. She wanted him to be their set designer for one of their operas in Germany. At first, he turned her down. "I wasn't willing to face a land that had tortured me," he said, but he couldn't get the offer out of his mind.

"It was a dream come true that I wouldn't have because my resentment kept me trapped. I decided that Germany was not going to control me any longer. I called Friedlinde back and told her I'd come." He struggled with his decision, explaining his conflict. "The Wagners supported Hitler," he said in a voice that still contained a hint of anguish. In the end, however, Milton decided he had to face these unpleasant truths rather than run from them.

In Germany, he remained conflicted. The work was exciting but being there triggered memories. He pushed the memories aside and focused on his work, but he couldn't push aside the language. "I resisted as much as I could, but there was no escaping it. I needed to direct the workers in what I wanted them to do." He found himself wondering if these same workers were among the Germans who had tortured him years earlier.

He learned the language so well that he was asked to become a German interpreter. "I told them absolutely not." He finally gave in and found that interpreting German gave him the courage to face his demons. "It brought me face to face with my own inner war. It forced me to face my fear." He clarified for me that when you're an interpreter, you can't just translate one word for another. You have to understand the people so you can understand the context of the language. "You have to be like a bridge, a bridge of understanding. You have to adopt the perceptions of those who speak the language," he explained. He then told me the lesson he learned; it took my breath away. "It forced me to understand people I didn't want to understand. It forced me to love people I had only known to fear. In doing that, I became free. It was my real release date from the German POW camp. If I hadn't done that, I'd still be imprisoned today."

I was speechless; "Wow" was all I could say. (Wow is my acronym for "With Out Words.") In my wordless beholdenment, I realized that beyond the heroism of living as a POW was the heroism required to make the post-POW journey, a heroism often not recognized or acknowledged. Finally, I spoke. "So the journey you made to become a German interpreter was your salvation."

He nodded.

"It was how you redeemed your suffering," I continued.

"Oh yes," he said with an almost childlike enthusiasm.

"It was how you met your Crescent Moon Bear," I cryptically added. Normally I would never speak of myths with patients, but here was a patient who *lived* mythical truths; I couldn't resist. "It's a myth about the journey after trauma . . . the journey to gather scattered pieces of broken self . . . the journey to meet the Great Compassionate Self paradoxically housed in the gruff, fearful self symbolized by a terrifying bear. The bear, however, houses the Great Compassionate Self and it is this part of our personhood with the energy to bring all the pieces of self back together so they can coexist peaceably."[5]

He laughed with recognition immediately. "You got it. That's it exactly. You know and understand the wisdom myths contain!"

"Not as much as I need to," I acknowledged. "It's taken me a long time to value and appreciate their hidden treasures. That's a story in itself."

"I don't suppose you know who Joseph Campbell is?" he asked.

"Are you kidding?" I responded. Everyone who watched Bill Moyers on the Public Broadcasting System knew the man who was probably the greatest mythologist of our time.

"Joe was my best friend," he said smiling. "I vacationed at his home in Hawaii," he said as he pulled out some watercolors of Hawaiian scenes. It was hard to contain my excitement as I heard tales of their adventures together. "Joe told me he and I travel in a forest without a path."

I looked at him quizzically.

" . . . We make our own trails," he said grinning.[6]

Understanding Trajectories 2 and 3: PTSD

Unlike Milton, about 20% to 30% of veterans are on trajectories 2 or 3. They have Posttraumatic Stress Disorder (PTSD).[7] *The Diagnostic and Statistical Manual of Mental Disorders* (DSM) is the fundamental reference for defining mental health. It identifies a con-

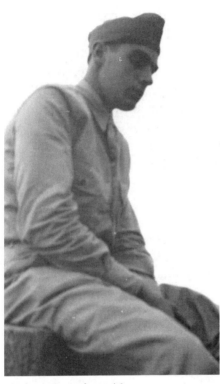

Milton Howarth, 1946.

stellation of symptoms that must be present for the diagnosis of PTSD.[8] These symptoms include: exposure to a traumatic event experienced with fear, helplessness, or horror; after the original trauma is over, the trauma is reexperienced through recollections, dreams, flashbacks, hallucinations, illusions, distress at cues that symbolize the trauma, or physiologic responses when confronted with cues reminiscent of the trauma. The distress of the reexperienced trauma causes people to exhibit avoidance behaviors and use emotional numbing in order to block out the trauma. In spite of their best efforts, however, there are times when the trauma is reexperienced anyway and the person exhibits symptoms of arousal such as: difficult sleep patterns, irritability or outbursts of anger, difficulty concentrating, hypervigilance (staying on guard and unable to calm down or relax), exaggerated startle response to noises or being touched. When these constellation of symptoms last for at least a month and cause significant impairment, a diagnosis of PTSD is made.[9]

Many people with PTSD have successfully suffered their war experiences by learning lessons that help them live their lives, deal with trauma, reckon with PTSD, and face their deaths. If they have received PTSD treatment, they can often tell me what helps them feel better. They might already have a network of friends with PTSD who can provide support. Family members usually know how to respond to breakthrough episodes of PTSD because it's familiar territory.

Other patients with PTSD have not had this experience. They've compartmentalized the trauma, banishing it into unconsciousness. They might have increased difficulty as death approaches and they become haunted by residual memories or corroding guilts. Others seem less affected.

When patients with PTSD are admitted to our Hospice and Palliative Care unit, they are sometimes anxious, suspicious, or angry. Leaving their homes to enter an unknown hospital environment is threatening, increasing their feelings of danger. The hospital environment itself can act as a trigger with its militarized processes. Their own anticipated death can act as a PTSD trigger. PTSD, especially when combined with alcohol abuse, has often taken its toll on their relationships, leaving much unfinished business to be resolved so a peaceful death can ensue. Sometimes they arrive at the end of their lives broken, bitterness poisoning their souls. However, it is never too late. As many of the stories in this book attest, opportunities for growth abound when death approaches and many people, even those who are bitter, avail themselves of the lessons.

I always ask combat veterans about their war experience: "Now is a time to look back over your life. Is there anything that might still be troubling you? Anything about the war that might still be haunting you?" I always sit quietly after these questions. These aren't the kind of answers you can hurry and they're not the kind of answers you just check off on an admission form.

Trajectory 2: Apparent Integration of Trauma

Some people seem to integrate trauma into their lives, but it emerges later when something unmasks the unresolved trauma. Though it might seem to come on suddenly after many years, a review of their lives usually finds it creeping out in subtle ways.

My theory is that people with delayed-onset PTSD have especially thick stoic walls. They have what I sometimes call "white

knuckle syndrome;" they hold on tightly. They've been able to successfully hide their symptoms. "I'm fine,"[10] becomes their shield to
keep others from suspecting what's beneath the surface. Because they
have effectively hidden their symptoms, PTSD has been difficult to
diagnose and treatment has been averted. Symptoms, however, leak
out in other ways: hollowness, aloofness, workaholism or its opposite
(job-hopping or joblessness), or addictions.

For those who have successfully hidden combat memories (even
from themselves), turmoil or agitation might surface at end of life
because as the conscious mind weakens with approaching death,
unconscious war memories sometimes surface. This delayed-onset
PTSD may be particularly overwhelming and frightening, requiring
intense support because these veterans have built especially strong
defensive walls. However, when they are able to push through their
defenses and summon the courage to recover scattered pieces of broken self, they can become role models for how to redeem suffering.
Ed is a good example. I met him in the Dying Healed course I teach.
The course is eight 2-hour/week classes for patients, staff, and volunteers throughout the hospital who want to learn principles of hospice and palliative care. Ed was an outpatient in the PTSD program.
He wanted to become a hospice volunteer.[11]

After the first class, Ed spoke with me. "You need to know I'm
here against my psychologist's advice. He says you'll probably be talking about death, which is going to trigger my PTSD. If I can't finish
the eight weeks, you'll know why."

Ed was able to stick out the first few classes that focus on managing symptoms and supporting patients' efforts to complete unfinished business so peacefulness can ensue. We then move into reckoning with our own unfinished business, realizing that if we don't
know how to touch our own anger, pain, fear, and guilt then we can't
help others reckon with theirs. This is a time when personal stories
often emerge, as did Ed's.

Ed was drafted after high school, and at first he was excited
about going to Vietnam. "That feeling lasted until the airplane I was
arriving in got shot at," he said. "That's when my confidence turned

to fear."

On his first mission, one of his comrades was killed. Ed was carrying the dead man's body back to their camp, but the Viet Cong were closing in on them so Ed had to leave his friend's body behind so they could retreat more quickly. He felt guilty for this in spite of the fact that it had been necessary to save lives.

Ed volunteered to go with the platoon sent back to retrieve his comrade's body. "We found him and brought him back, but I've never been able to shake the guilt," he said. Afterwards, he began drinking. "I had never been one to drink before, but after that day, I did. It helped drown out the fear and guilt—besides, everyone else was doing it."

The class of about 20 people sat spellbound, receiving a first-hand account of lessons warriors learn.

"It changed my relationships with people too," Ed resumed. "I felt I couldn't depend on anyone except myself now. I had to be in control. I always volunteered to be the point man on patrol; I hated to be in the rear." Further experiences in combat continued to traumatize him. Hit by shrapnel, he spent four weeks in a Saigon hospital. He was then sent back into battle. When one of his comrades was killed by a mortar round, Ed went out to pull him back to cover. "When I grabbed his ankles to drag his body, his legs came off in my hands."

The whole room gasped in collective horror when we heard this part of his story. Ed jumped ahead to the ending of his story. "My year was up and I flew home. There was a girl selling flowers in the airport. I didn't pay any attention to her until she came up to me and spit on my uniform."

He spent the next eight months lying on the beach and drinking, trying to forget everything. Then he felt ready to pick up his life. He stopped drinking, got married, found a job in a factory. For years, he thought everything was fine. He had nightmares about Vietnam, but rarely thought consciously about it.

He had acquired habits he didn't associate with the war: he was often jumpy, he got panic attacks when he was taking his car through a car wash, and he stopped going to church because the music pounded in his head. Still, he managed to function fairly well and did not realize that these were symptoms of PTSD. Then 25 years later, he needed surgery on his knee; the shrapnel still there was creating infection and blood clots. The doctors said they might have to amputate the leg. "All I could think about was that man's legs coming off in my hands in Vietnam. That's when I lost it. Nothing they did could calm me down. They finally sent a psychiatrist who diagnosed me with PTSD." He had begun to get treatment, but was still struggling with his PTSD. "I still can't shake the guilt from my first mission when I had to leave my buddy behind."

Ed stopped, looking at the class expectantly. He was through telling his story, but I was still recovering from its impact. Slowly I gathered my wits about me. I suggested that he write a letter to his buddy asking for forgiveness for having to leave him behind.

"My psychologist already had me do that and it didn't help," he responded matter-of-factly.

"All right," I said. "Then how about having your comrade write you a letter?"

Ed looked at me incredulously. "I told you—he *died!*"

"I realize that," I said. "But if your buddy were in this room hearing everything you've been saying, how do you think he'd respond? Write his response in a letter that starts out 'Dear Ed.' Write it from his perspective. Use 'I' not 'he'."

Ed seemed skeptical but agreed to try it.

The next week he returned to class brandishing his letter, eager to share its contents. The letter he had his buddy write to him was filled with understanding and forgiveness, the understanding and forgiveness that Ed was finally ready to give himself. "It really helped," he told the class. "I feel free—like a new person."

He looked like a new person too. His posture was straighter, his face lighter.

"This letter is like a 'Get out of Jail Free' card," I remarked after hearing its liberating contents and seeing its transforming results.

"It really is," Ed said quietly. "This is *my* independence day. This marks the day I've been freed from the prison that my guilt has held me in all these years."

The entire class sat in amazement. We were beholding a hero's journey, a journey that brought new hope for Ed's life. Now that his trauma had been integrated, he wanted to help others. He began volunteering on our Hospice unit daily and has done so for more than seven years. "I'm not going to leave these vets behind," he told us.

Veterans on Trajectory 3: Unresolved PTSD

Unlike Ed, some veterans who have served in dangerous assignments struggle with PTSD shortly after the trauma occurs. The part of themselves that experienced trauma gets locked up. Such was the case with Raymond. He was in a local hospital with end-stage liver disease, the result of excessive alcohol usage used to self-medicate his PTSD he sustained with the Vietnam War. His doctor phoned me, requesting admission for the patient to our Hospice and Palliative Care unit.

I had a mental image of what Raymond probably looked like based on his diagnosis: swollen abdomen due to accumulated fluid, mentally dull from built-up toxins, and the ruddy, disheveled appearance of a man who no longer took pride in himself.

That night, I dreamed I went to meet Raymond, and he arose from his hospital bed, tall, handsome and well-groomed, in a three-piece business suit. Then I awoke, puzzled by my dream. Raymond arrived later that day; he looked sick and ungroomed like I had expected.

The hospice and palliative care team held a meeting at his bedside to learn more about Raymond. He told us he had PTSD and had been a drifter since Vietnam, finding it difficult to establish relationships or maintain a job for long periods. "I don't know what got into me. I wasn't raised like that. I should have done something with my life," he told us. I asked him if there was anything from the war that might still be troubling him.

"I try not to think about it," he said. "But what keeps coming back is the eyes of my comrades. I saw peace in the eyes of the dead; I saw fear in the eyes of the living." Our team sat in stunned silence as we let ourselves experience war vicariously.

Later in my office, I kept reflecting on the profundity of this casual comment and the detachedness with which it was said. I let its chilling truth penetrate my illusory, warless world. Now I understood the meaning of my dream. It was not this Raymond I had seen, but the Raymond he might have been. I had met the Raymond who had not gone to Vietnam. That's when I realized that war robs people of many things, but possibly the most significant is a young person's hope and dreams.

Heroes are veterans like Milton, Ed, and Raymond who are able to make the courageous journey to redeem the suffering war inflicted. Some might hail Milton more of a hero than the other two because of the profound wisdom he had. Some might hail Ed the most heroic because he redeemed his suffering through volunteering. Raymond might not be called a hero at all because he got lost in alcoholism and failed to recover from it; his heroism came from sacrificing the life he *could have had.*

Families Also Suffer the Effects of War

Heroes go into dark places and find light. Having listened to hundreds of stories from veterans and their families, I've come to appreciate how much darkness both veterans *and their families* have endured and how much light they've borne as they find their way back from war. Families of combat veterans are often unsung heroes; these include families who have had to bear the death of a loved one in battle as well as those who have survived but returned fundamentally changed.[12]

I end presentations that I do about veterans by having the veterans in the audience stand so the audience can honor them. Then I have family members stand if they have sustained the physical or emotional loss of a loved one due to war. This is important because it validates the influence that the military has had on family members. Mike, a chaplain at Tidewell Hospice, told me how much this helped him. "For 40 years, I've been in congregations that acknowledged veterans on Veteran's Day; but this is the first time anyone has acknowledged me and what my family went through." Mike's brother had been killed in Vietnam. He spoke about how healing it was to be able to bring his grief into the open and talk about it with colleagues. As a result, the hospice he worked for started a remarkable program to support military families.[13]

Our Hospice and Palliative Care program uses a simple angel pin to acknowledge family sacrifice. The angel's dress is an American flag. We ceremonially pin it on family members who tell us about the hardships they have experienced due to the military's impact on their loved one or on themselves. These sacrifices can take many forms.

Roles in military families can be conflicted when there are frequent deployments. The civilian partner runs the household in the military member's absence. The military partner returns, and either feels "lost because I'm not needed" or resumes control of the household and the civilian partner feels "pushed aside. After all, I've been doing this the whole time he/she's been gone."

Wives sometimes complain that their veteran husband trivializes problems that the wife is having. "He's seen horrible things so he just laughs when I tell him things I'm going through. It makes me mad, but at the same time, he's right. My problems are small compared to war. Now I feel guilty if I complain about anything."

If the soldier has PTSD, it affects entire family systems and generations of families. Relationships change in expected and unexpected ways after war. "After he came back, he had to know where I was every minute of the day. He had to know I was safe. He was never like that before," a patient's wife complained. A mother told me, "I didn't know the person who came back after the war. We had a stranger in our midst; we still do." Another patient's sister said, "Most of my brother stayed over there in that war. He never really came home." One of my patients told me, "I've been fighting that war every day since I returned home." His wife interrupted him saying, "You mean *we've* been fighting that war every day." In one way or another, the soldier changes after war and their relationships with others can never be the same. Much of a family's suffering surrounds grieving the loss these changes cause. Helping families come to peace with their changed loved one usually involves helping them grieve so they can let go of how their prewar family member was and open up to a new relationship that includes the changes that their relationship incurs. It means letting go of old expectations and exploring ways to birth new expectations within relationships.

Family members may feel angry because of the veteran's detached façade, angry outbursts, or overprotective behaviors. "The wall he hides behind takes a long time to come down and can go back up in an instant," one wife said frustratedly. Family members often appreciate receiving explanations about PTSD because it provides new meaning and context for behaviors they may not have previously understood to be related to combat. "That explains so much," they sometimes say as they look back on their lives together with new insight after they're told about PTSD. Sometimes they feel guilty that they hadn't previously understood combat's impact on their loved one. Conversely, some family members might be desensitized to the trauma or tired of hearing about it. They might be angry with how much of the veteran's life is spent living in the past; they don't want to hear about PTSD. Also, dealing with PTSD sometimes leaves wives isolated without a support system; they might be exhausted from caregiver burden if the veteran's PTSD escalates prior to death which it sometimes does. Sometimes family members don't have much left to give by the time the veteran is admitted to our Hospice and Palliative Care unit.

The aftermath of war can leave other kinds of trauma that affect families, for example sterility or birth defects from Agent Orange or other chemicals used in warfare. "I live with Vietnam every day. My daughter has spina bifida," one woman told me. Silence about the war can affect relationships. "There's this whole part of him he won't let me see. This is a part of him I want to love, but he won't let me," a rueful wife told me.

On the other hand, some wives don't want to know; they're

afraid. This was the case with Tommy Bill's wife, Judy. I had sent him the manuscript of this book so he could review his story for accuracy; Judy read it too. Though he had previously given her his diary, Judy hadn't read it. "I didn't want to see him as someone who went through that kind of stuff," she said. Her decision was based on wanting to focus on the "smiling" Tommy. "I just didn't want to see the other Tommy; it hurt too much to know what he had been through." Tommy says Judy is now reading his diary and asking him questions. He e-mailed me about how this is changing their relationship. "This has opened up her eyes and opened up another special place in our relationship!!!"

Tommy says that he's still trying to figure out what to tell the rest of his family about what he's been through. "I had only told them about how beautiful the country was. I had made light of the dangers and told them that what I was doing was like camping out in south Florida." I can only anticipate the "special place" that will be created in Tommy's relationship with his family when they learn the truth. It will no doubt help to set him free.

Some Needed Clarifications about PTSD

It's important to reemphasize that not all combat veterans who have been traumatized experience PTSD, and that having some of the symptoms of PTSD after returning home from war is normal. It's when the symptoms persist and cause significant distress or impairment that PTSD is then diagnosed. It's also important to remember that not all combat veterans have been traumatized. Surprisingly, some combat assignments expose their participants to little combat and are considered relatively safe.

On the other hand, I hope my emphasis on combat veterans doesn't discount how non-combat veterans have suffered effects of the military culture. Dangerous missions are required for numerous military assignments. In fact, sometimes I think the trauma they sustain can be even more damaging because it often goes unacknowledged or is minimized because "he didn't see combat." Indeed, noncombat military deaths occurred in more than 18,000 Korean-era veterans, 42,000 Vietnam-era veterans, and 2,000 Gulf War-era veterans.[14] All veterans set aside prime years in their lives, delayed personal goals, separated from loved ones, and went to strange and sometimes dangerous parts of the world. They were expected to do difficult jobs they may or may not have been inclined to perform, all the while "grinning and bearing it" or "biting the bullet." All were trained to defend their country and be willing to risk their lives if necessary to do so. Most of us declined those "opportunities."

My emphasis on some of the harmful effects of military culture, however, in no way negates the many beneficial effects. "The military was the best thing that ever happened to me," is something I hear frequently. Military life brought order and structure to chaotic teenage lives that sometimes badly needed order and structure. Communal living helped them feel "belonged" and gave them a sense of teamwork and service for someone other than themselves. Educational opportunities during and after service often abound. There is no doubt that the military has provided many beneficial effects to those who've served in its ranks.

I hope I haven't slighted Korean or World War II veterans because I've disproportionately highlighted Vietnam veterans. Because World War II veterans were treated as heroes, their sacrifices have at least been acknowledged. I had a World War II veteran ask me why I validated the suffering of Vietnam veterans more than other war veterans. "My validating the Vietnam veterans' suffering in no way diminishes what you did," I told him. "It just acknowledges what they did *not* get." He seemed satisfied, expressing understanding with the distinction.

There has not been much emphasis on PTSD with wars prior to Vietnam because it was not recognized as an official diagnosis until 1980. But that doesn't mean it didn't exist or may not have been as prevalent. Previous generations called it "battle fatigue" or "shell shock." Writings as far back as the Bible even reference symptoms of PTSD, though it was not recognized as such.[15]

There are probably several reasons I emphasize the suffering of

Vietnam veterans. No doubt there are personal reasons that reflect my own healing, not to mention that Vietnam was a war of my own generation. Beyond the personal reasons, I can't ignore what I see; unresolved combat issues surface as veterans die. Vietnam remains a gaping wound for our nation. Likewise, I can't write about what I've not seen, which is the case of Gulf War and the Afghanistan and Iraq War veterans. Their stories will no doubt be the same and different; war has universal and unique effects on people.

I went to a lecture by an Iraq War veteran who spoke about the PTSD he suffered. He said he slept with a gas mask at his bedside. "When I wake up terrorized in the middle of the night by dreams of invisible gas, I put it over my face so I know I'm safe. I know this is irrational, but it works," he had said.

As I listened, I couldn't help but wonder how hospice interventions will need to change to accommodate "invisible" enemy poisons. What will the next generation of hospice nurses need to know in order to respond to these veterans' sufferings?

Indeed, the VA intends to learn all it can about veterans' needs at the end of life so it can respond. Congress passed a law stating all enrolled veterans must have access to hospice care.[16] This means that every enrolled veteran (regardless of category or service-connection) is eligible to receive hospice and palliative care provided or purchased by the VA. The VA has accepted this responsibility so we can provide leadership to the nation. I hope that Veteran Service Organizations will advocate on the veteran's behalf to assure the entitlement veterans are due. "Death with honor" has been a code the military has lived by. It's a code that is supposed to be maintained after they leave the military.

I also hope people won't think all those with PTSD are condemned to a difficult death. In fact, they sometimes have a better death. PTSD can be a complicating factor; it can also be a redeeming factor. I'm often struck by their resiliency and the many ways that in spite of what they've been through, they've been able to laugh, relate, find hope, share, and stay connected. They have been victims, but they've also been survivors. Many learn to live from a deeper part within themselves.

Some experts say that PTSD is a normal response to an abnormal situation and that anyone who experiences war and can remain untouched may be abnormal. Others, however, say just the opposite; they don't believe PTSD to be a valid threat to mental health. I read a newspaper article calling PTSD a "national enfeeblement" that is breeding a country of people too fragile to handle their feelings and faults so that they become incompetent to handle trauma and "can't cope with life unassisted."[17] The author sees PTSD as eroding the stoicism, self-reliance, and courage the country was founded on. I think this opinion is both harmful and helpful. Keeping the effects of war silent behind stoic walls minimizes society having to deal with it, but I wonder how many veterans with PTSD (or their families) would agree with the author's naïve opinion? Broad generalizations have interfered with people appropriately receiving treatment for PTSD. I've seen similar sweeping statements made about people with other disruptions in mental health, such as depression. "They'd be fine if they'd just snap out of it and use a little will power to get things done." Mental health is incompletely understood and its resultant stigma keeps people from seeking treatment.

I've seen veterans and families receive comfort in finding out about PTSD, to know it has a name and there's help. At the same time, I think it wise to be cautious about viewing someone with PTSD as permanently damaged. No matter how traumatic an experience has been and how deeply wounded a person is, people with PTSD survive and thrive. We have to be careful about medicalizing trauma *and* we have to be careful about pretending it's not there or ignoring it or denying it when it is—or worse stigmatizing them by labeling them an "enfeeblement" so that they feel weak and ashamed.

We also have to be careful about casting protestors of war as villains. They, too, were sometimes jailed and ostracized for their beliefs. Many felt betrayed because the soldiers that they were speaking up for and trying to help were the ones who cursed and spat on them.

There are other difficult issues surrounding PTSD that contaminate diagnosis and treatment, the most notable being financial compensation. Disability payments sometimes cause people to fake or exaggerate symptoms of PTSD. For example, we were medicating a patient according to the medications listed that he had taken at home, yet he was excessively sedated. His sister shed some light on why. "He doesn't take any of those medications the PTSD clinic sends him. The meds are still in the original mailers. He just wanted them to think he had PTSD so he could get his monthly check for it."

This kind of fraud not only costs the taxpayers millions of dollars, it adversely affects people who legitimately have PTSD. I admitted a patient who clearly had suffered PTSD most of his postwar life. He was aware of PTSD and that help was available. When I asked him why he hadn't availed himself, he said, "There are too many veterans who fake PTSD symptoms to get disability checks from the government. I don't want to be associated with them." Each time I hear veterans say these kinds of statements, I feel sad. I wonder if veterans who fake PTSD know how much damage they do to their fellow veterans who have PTSD, or to their own integrity, for that matter.

I've also occasionally seen practitioners cast all who have PTSD into the "faking" category—just like I used to do as I described in Chapter 2 when I met Tommy Bills. My hope is that practitioners will find a way to discern the difference so those with PTSD can receive treatment and those who do not can have their claims revoked.

I hope people will not think me an expert in PTSD; I'm not. All of my observations about PTSD are within the context of dying people. There are thousands of articles written about PTSD; none talk about how PTSD affects dying, leaving me to my own speculations. I have no way of knowing how valid my observations are when applied to those who are not imminently dying. I think dying veterans might teach us a way to learn and appreciate PTSD in ways we've not previously known. Dying veterans may shed light on ways to intervene earlier in the trauma cycle. For example, some PTSD programs don't allow dying patients into their groups because it triggers trauma for the other participants. However, a dying veteran might allow the opportunity for the rest of the group to go into the trauma openly in a safe and supported environment so that interventions can be provided before each person has to face their death. Avoiding dealing with it, might be a reason I see so much of it at end of life.

I hope the *Diagnostic and Statistical Manual* (DSM) will address PTSD in people who are dying. The DSM identifies how PTSD expresses itself differently in children. Children's dreams may be "frightening without recognizable content" or "trauma-specific reenactment may occur."[18] In my experience, dying people often express PTSD as children do; they act it out. I hope the DSM will address PTSD in the dying so attention and information can be provided in this context.

My writing about PTSD is strictly anecdotal. I hope the anecdotes have been provocative so research will be stimulated. Many of the standard treatments for PTSD are not feasible when patients are imminently dying. Many drugs usually taken for PTSD are no longer able to be administered by mouth and are unavailable by other routes. Normal "talk therapy" or groups are not practical. Usual "grounding techniques" may not be effective because the person's rational access to his conscious mind is limited.

Research might help us anticipate when PTSD might occur so we can proactively intervene. Many questions surround the emergence of PTSD at the end of life. Right now, we don't know how often it surfaces to complicate the dying process. I also don't know the qualitative relationship between stoicism and a "good" death. Sometimes I wonder if the strength of a veteran's stoic wall to encapsulate, segregate, and isolate them from healing resources within the self might be a risk factor for developing PTSD.

I don't know the answers to these questions, but I'd like to. We are still learning how to help dying people who have PTSD. We are gradually coming to understand the lifetime effects of war. I hope we will continue to develop that knowledge; if we don't, we have failed these men and women in a very human and fundamental way.

Finding Peace

I used to assume that combat soldiers liked war, but experience has taught me otherwise. Soldiers know that war is hell; many return from war bearing no firearms. Instead, they bear peace within themselves, with others, with the world, with God. Their souls have borne enough war; they dare to live in the world without it.

Others are unable to bear peace, but that doesn't mean that they don't yearn for it. Though some came away from war with a violent nature, beyond the fierce veneer I often discovered a gentle core that desperately longed for peace. It seems paradoxical that these men and women who fought for peace, sometimes find so little for themselves, even resisting recovery programs. I hope they can find it within themselves to summon the courage to seek effective treatment.

The reason some veterans don't seek treatment is because they feel betrayed by the government; they often don't trust a government agency's help. A national agency run by veterans, *The Vet Center,* offers information and programs for veterans with PTSD.[19] Not only do staff at the *Vet Centers* have the expertise and resources to deal with the trauma, but they can provide outreach services to the 85% of veterans who are not enrolled in the VA. I hope all combat veterans will avail themselves of their services.

Sometimes, PTSD surfaces for the first time at end of life and is particularly frightening at a time when the patient is especially vulnerable. I hope that hospice organizations and *Vet Centers* will partner to develop "PTSD Response Teams" that can respond to this emergency when it surfaces at end of life; certainly, no single nurse or other hospice staff member should be expected to handle this alone.

I hope no one will let stoicism, denial, stigma, ignorance, or fear keep them from seeking information and support so that PTSD does not continue to squeeze them out of their own lives. One reason I think it is so important to help veterans at the end of life is because it is one last opportunity to help them find peace before they leave their earthly journey.

Those veterans that find peace offer hope to the rest of us. Up to 84% of all people experience a traumatic event at some time during their lives.[20] It is not unusual for PTSD to develop after someone has been the victim of a crime, abuse, or a natural disaster. We can apply fundamental lessons we've learned from combat to non-combat trauma. Though I've not been traumatized in the way combat veterans have, my soul has been tried in other ways. I've come to appreciate that just as suffering is part of the human condition, PTSD-like symptoms often accompany suffering at least for awhile. As a civilian, veterans have also shown me how I hide behind my own stoic wall. They've shown me my own fighting/flighting/freezing behaviors; in truth, we are *all* "wounded warriors" with our own inner wars.

I've also come to realize that we can stop outer wars by learning how to stop inner wars. It's difficult to acknowledge that wars created on a national level are a reflection of the battles we create within ourselves. Even more difficult is being willing to confront the hostile self in each of us that creates those wars; we self-righteously pray for peace while we perpetuate the illusion that we are not contributing to its lack.

I experienced this myself recently. I was flying home from a speaking tour. I sat in the window seat on the plane. Next to me was a man with his arm protruding about a foot into my space. I politely pointed this out to him. He grunted and retracted his elbow, but only slightly. I told him that we'd need to share the armrest and I placed my elbow on it; he didn't budge. Now it was no longer about comfort and armrests; it had turned into a power struggle. For the next 10 minutes I plotted ways to get back at him. I saw him look up from his reading to stare out the window for a time; I strongly considered pulling the shade down. His wife sat opposite him, and their conversation indicated that they had a lot of money; I considered ways to use this information. I could chide him for his sense of entitlement when he sits in the coach section or I could ridicule him for not being rich enough to sit in first class where he'd have all the elbow room he needed; but then I felt a sneeze coming on. This too could prove useful. I could refrain from covering my mouth. Just the previous week there had been a story on the news about an airline passenger with TB; maybe I could tell Mr. Elbow I had TB. I settled on sneezing, but the satisfaction I began to feel from my revenge suddenly melted as I realized what I was doing. I laughed as I realized what a hypocrite I was. Here I was running around the country talking about the effect of our personal wars on national wars, and I'm sitting here plotting World War III against an elbow!

"This is how it all starts," I told myself, a little less smugly than I do when I lecture.

Lessons about War

- Combat soldiers don't usually fight for themselves; they are mostly selflessly motivated to fight for a cause and to fight for comrades.
- Each war was different. Each had its own culture that exerted a different influence on young soldiers.
- Ask questions about combat history sensitively; be willing to hear what others don't want to hear. Pay attention to the relationship between combat history, postcombat integration of trauma (or its lack), and the quality of death (turmoil vs. serenity).
- Conceptualizing combat-traumatized veterans along three trajectories is an overly-simplified, but helpful, way to understand the aftermath of war: 1) true integration and healing of postwar trauma, 2) *apparent* integration of combat trauma with the veteran *seemingly* unscathed until combat memories escape from behind stoic walls as they face personal illness, death, or some other trigger, and 3) incomplete integration of trauma (PTSD).
- Heroes go into dark places and find light. Veterans *and their families* have endured much darkness and they've borne much light as they find their way back from war.
- Acknowledge the hardships that military families have gone through.
- Use the information in Appendix D to understand the unique considerations for providing bereavement care to veterans and their

families. If you are a hospice organization, let Tidewell Hospice inspire you to start a program for families of veterans.

- Reach out to *Vet Centers* in your community to get help for vets struggling with PTSD. If you are a hospice organization, partner with a *Vet Center* in your community to provide services to veterans who have PTSD, especially if it is emerging for the first time or is complicating a veteran's death. Go to: www.vetcenter.va.gov and www.ncptsd.org for more information about PTSD.
- If you have been the victim of crime, abuse, natural disaster, etc., recognize that you, too, might be struggling with PTSD. Reach out for help. Don't let trauma squeeze you out of your own life.
- We stop outer wars by learning how to stop inner wars sometimes.
- Sometimes war robs people of many things, but possibly the most significant is a young person's hope and dreams.
- Soldiers know that war is hell; many return from war bearing no firearms. Instead, they bear peace within themselves, with others, with the world, with God. Their souls have borne enough war; they dare to live in the world without it.
- It is important to help veterans at the end of life because it is one last opportunity to help them find peace before they leave their earthly journey.

Chapter Five

"I Was a Soldier. I Am a Soldier. I Will Always Be a Soldier."

When the power of love
Overcomes the love of power
Then, and only then,
Shall we have peace.
—Anonymous
(Bulletin board in the
DaNang Red Cross Center, Freedom Hill)[1]

Veterans' identity can persist long after discharge from military service. This sense of belonging can be rekindled when they come to the VA. There's camaraderie between patients who are no longer strangers once they meet inside VA walls. Hospitalizations sometimes seem like reunions among people who have never before met. Commonly, I've taken phone calls from families or hospice workers who tell me of someone who "wants to come to the VA to die." Maybe the camaraderie provides a sense of security that makes it easier to let go of earthly attachments. I recently experienced this personally with a friend of mine.

Shortly after I married, I had become close friends with Memrie,[2] a career-military nurse. She owned a boat, and it was on her dock that I had cleaned those 50 or 60 fish so I could acclimate myself to blood and guts on my first step toward becoming a nurse (Chapter 1). Though she was my mother's age, she had made strikingly different decisions. Never married, she had served in World War II, Korea, and Vietnam taking care of "my boys," as she affectionately called them.

Memrie moved to another city a few hours away, but we

remained in contact for over 35 years. At age 91, she had been independent and in good health until she suffered a heart attack. My husband and I went to be with her in the hospital. She was weak and
confused, not recognizing us initially. We told a few fishing stories
from the old days and her memory sparked.

"You're a nurse aren't you Deborah?" she said, fighting for her
recollections, apologizing for its gaps. "The VA, right?"

"You're right, Memrie. The VA," I said crawling into bed with
her, laying my head on her shoulder and putting my arm around her.
"Is it okay if I get in bed with you?"

"Yeah. It feels good," she said, patting my arm. She was weak
and her words were difficult to understand. We told stories from
when we had been neighbors. She had retired as a Lieutenant
Colonel in the Air Force, and I had been having babies. Some things
she said made sense; others didn't. It made her mad. "I just don't
understand why my mind won't think right," she'd say.

"Well I like your mind 'not thinking right'," I said light-heartedly. "It makes me feel right at home because mine hasn't been thinking too good since menopause myself."

We talked about dying. She said she wasn't afraid to die; she was
ready. She said she had spoken with her pastor; she told me she could
feel her mother near.

"Mama Lou," I responded with fond recollection. "She's coming
to escort you home no doubt," I answered.

Then she told me she wanted to go to the VA to die. "That's
where I belong," she said. Normally I'd have thought the same, but
I knew she only had a day or so to live. The trip would be too difficult. I had spoken with her nephew and family who lived nearby;
they wanted her close to them in her final days.

"I wish that could happen too," I said snuggling in close to her.
"You're too weak to make the trip, Memrie. It would be too hard for
you now. That's why I'm here. The VA came to you."

She relaxed in my arms. I began to massage her back. It was not
a short, jerky-motioned massage; rather, it was long, slow, easing
movements of my hands, fingertips never leaving her skin. Through

it all she kept repeating, "Oh, that feels so good."

"Think about all those soldiers you've nursed, Memrie. You called them 'your boys'," I whispered. "They're all here; they're all thanking you for the care you gave them; they're all saluting you and waiting for you to come home with them. It's your time, Memrie. Go on home to be with your boys." She relaxed, nodding that she understood. I kept massaging, occasionally urging her on with, "Let go. Open up. It's okay. Relax."

Memrie died the next day. After the funeral, her nephew gave me her dog tags. "She would have wanted you to have them," he said. I wanted to have them too.

I've always found women veterans like Memrie interesting. I think about the culture of 1940s America when women were encouraged to be housewives and silently support their husbands. Yet, here were women who defied the culture, sometimes even their parents and peers. They marched off to join the ranks and not in small numbers either. More than 400,000 women served during World War II.[3] These women often have a strength and sense of self that cause me to compare their constitutions to my own at that age, an age when I was busy trying to please and conform. These women were cast from a very different mold.

Women veterans have other stories, too. One of the consequences of being immersed in a male culture is an increased incidence of sexual assault. Several years ago, a national television show did a story about sexual assault in the military.[4] There was a call-in number for women to identify their needs so the VA could provide follow-up care. I helped staff the phones that night. Timidly and tearfully, women hesitantly told me their stories of pain and violation, shame, and silence. "I thought I had put it behind me," one said to me. "I didn't realize that some of the things I've experienced over the past 15 years have been related to feeling so powerless, not only while I was assaulted, but afterward. At that time there was no one I could report it to because there would have been repercussions." The symptoms they suffered were yet another reminder that PTSD is not limited to combat.

As with male veterans, women experience a deep bond with their fellow comrades. I saw this with a patient who came to us with severe end-stage dementia. She didn't speak to anyone, no longer even recognizing her family; we were mute to her world, and she seemed mute to ours. We sometimes sat her in a chair in the hallway facing our aquarium where she numbly watched the fish. One afternoon a volunteer came down the hallway. "I know her," Maxine said with surprise. "She's a Marine Corps veteran from the same Women's Marine Association I belong to!"

Maxine walked up to the patient's chair and gustily greeted her in the lingo of the Marines. "Semper Fi!" she said.

Our mute patient straightened her wilted frame and directed a piercing gaze at Maxine. With a smile we'd never seen and a purposefulness we'd not known her to possess, the patient reached out to shake her comrade's hand. "Semper Fi," she responded. It caused everyone in the busy hallway to pause; another soldier had just been brought home.

Gratitude

A sense of belonging helps soldiers come back home; gratitude helps as well. I was lowering the flag in my front yard to half-mast the day after the *Challenger* space shuttle exploded. Surprisingly, I found myself a bit angry. Later that day our hospital was going to have a Memorial Service for all the veterans who had died in the past four months at the medical center. I found myself wondering, "Why aren't we lowering the flags for them? Their contributions are no less important."

I have had similar feelings about military certificates we posted above each patient's bed. An official-looking document, it cites the veteran's name, years served in the military, and the seal of the branch of service to which they had belonged. Prominently featured are the words, "We appreciate our Veterans."

When I first saw these certificates, I thought, "Is this really going to matter? This is too little, too late." I was wrong. Repeatedly, my patients told me how proud they were to have these posted over their beds. I realized then how military service was and remained a source of pride and identity for many veterans. It had shaped their lives; it had formed their young adult identity, and it continued to exert its influence. The certificates are also important to families. They often want to frame them, especially after the veteran dies.

"Thank you for serving our country" is a small thing to say, but it can make a big impact. It requires sincerity, however; words become trite and perfunctory when they don't come from personal exploration and development of awareness of the sacrifices veterans have made. Veterans often downplay that sacrifice saying, "I just did what needed to be done," or "others did more than I did."

Now each time I post a certificate, I reach out to shake the veteran's hand. I tell them I appreciate their service. Some shrug it off nonchalantly. For many others, a chord is struck, tears well, chins quiver. Over and over, I hear "No one's ever said that to me before" or "I didn't know anyone cared anymore" or "Thank you. It means so much that you haven't forgotten."

I often confess my vulnerability of forgetting: "These certificates are as much for me as they are for you. Sometimes, I *do* forget. Sometimes, I take you for granted. I don't want to do that."

After the success of the certificates, we purchased American flag lapel pins that said "Honored Veteran." Carrying a supply in my white lab coat pocket, I had a convenient tool that symbolized gratitude. After speaking about their military service, I ceremonially pin them on patients. "Each time you look at this pin, may you know how much I appreciate *my* freedom. I know that it comes with a price and that you helped pay that price."

The VA also contracts with private nursing homes to provide care for veterans. VA nurses regularly visit the veterans under these VA contracts to assure they're receiving appropriate care. I gave a supply of flag lapel pins to one of the nurses, Brenda. She met with a patient who was in the dining room of a community nursing home. When she finished her assessment, she pinned a flag on his shirt, thanking him for his service. A patient at a nearby table said, "I'm a veteran too. Can I have one of those?" Five other veterans, overhearing him, chimed in.

"It was amazing," Brenda later told me. "They started swapping military stories. They hadn't realized they were each veterans. I left an hour later and they were still sharing their stories." The nursing home staff was so impressed that they started regular groups for their veterans and created programs to honor them on Veterans Day and Memorial Day. This has been especially important for the veterans who have received care for years at the VA and sometimes feel abandoned when they were later placed in a nursing home for care. "The pin reminds them that they still belong to the community of veterans," Brenda said.

We also express gratitude for military service during our Quality of Life (QOL) rounds with patients. QOL rounds are weekly bedside meetings we do with all our patients. We use rolling chairs to gather at the bedside. QOL rounds bring a conscious intention to be *with* patients and their families. QOL is not easy when we're so busy doing things to patients and for patients. Our team has found that soulfully listening to patients' stories allows us privileged witness to their lives. In the process, relationships are deepened and patients feel loved and supported on their journey. Team members are, likewise, touched and changed by the patients.

Expressing gratitude often precipitates some amazing stories. Our QOL team was sitting at the bedside of Mr. Black, a World War II veteran who had served in Germany. We expressed our gratitude to him for the sacrifices he had made. He didn't say anything, but tears welled up in his eyes. We waited, abiding his feelings with him. Then I asked him how his war experiences had molded and shaped his life.

He thought carefully for a moment before answering. "It's never left me. It's never gone, especially the children."

We looked at him quizzically, not sure what he meant.

"Every day, I still see the starving German children scrounging through garbage cans. I can't get their images out of my mind," he said, tearfully. "I fought for *them*."

We sat in silence, providing emotional space for his trauma and grief while vicariously allowing ourselves to abide with his perspective on war.

A pharmacy intern, Ursula, was sitting in on the meeting as part of her training. The team knew little about Ursula beyond her name, adding to the impact of what she was about to say. She quietly rose from her seat and drew close to the patient. "I want to thank you for what you did for those children," she said earnestly. "I want to thank you for my father." She took a deep breath while we sat startled in suspended animation. Then she continued. "He was one of those starving German children. Because of what you did to help him, he decided that when he grew up, he would raise his children in America. I'm here because of you." The patient could only cry and the team could only sit in stunned amazement.

Though I could cite hundreds of stories that highlight the importance of gratitude, there have also been times when gratitude was not welcomed. "Thanks for what?" one veteran asked me. "Shooting people? Cowering in my foxhole unable to move? Burning peoples' homes?" He made me realize that offering gratitude can be meaningless unless we understand that soldier's story.

It's Never too Late to Say "I'm Sorry"

For some veterans, gratitude is not enough; some veterans need an apology. In the early 1990s, the Persian Gulf War veterans were returning home victorious, greeted as heroes. For some of our Vietnam vets, this was a bitter reminder of how differently *they* had been greeted. "No one ever welcomed us home like that," Larry told me. "They didn't want to see 'Nam vets or hear what we had to say." He was glad that new veterans didn't have to suffer what he had suffered. "But it still hurts," he added. I could feel the bitterness that was still poisoning his life thirty years later. Then he said something that was heartbreaking. "All that for nothing. My buddies killed for nothing. The government duped us. It was all just politics and money. Our nation is sinful. All I've been through these past years since the war . . . for nothing."

I let myself feel his bitterness, then I rose slowly and knelt before his chair. I took his hands in mine, forced my gaze to meet his hung head and downcast eyes. I felt the shame of our nation's shabby treatment of vets like Larry. I let myself feel the bitterness of suffering in vain, the emptiness of suffering without meaning. Then I spoke words he needed to hear. "Larry, I am so sorry for how we treated you. I am so sorry for the indignities you've had to suffer because of our ignorance. I don't know if that war was an unjust one or not. If it was, then you've had to bear the 'sins' of our nation. What I *do* know, is that you were treated unjustly. I want you to know that you are a hero. And unsung heroes are the most worthy kind."

His eyes never diverted from mine, then he slumped forward in my arms and sobbed.

I realized several things that day. Whether we win a war or not, whether a war is just or unjust, does not change what soldiers went through, the sacrifices they made. In fact, losing wars or fighting in wars they come to believe are unjust make the sacrifices that much more difficult to bear.

A colleague of mine, Lorraine, had a similar experience. She was in a waiting room at a doctor's office. She overheard a conversation of another patient with the receptionist about insurance. After he sat down, she asked if he was a veteran; he acknowledged he was. "Have you ever gone to the VA for your medical needs?" she asked.

"Others need it more than me," he told her.

She told him because of his service to his country, he had earned the care and might be eligible to receive it. "I don't feel that way because when I returned from Vietnam, I was cursed, spat upon, and called a murderer," he said. In a voice cracking with emotion, he added, "I was made to feel like I didn't deserve *anything*."

Lorraine leaned forward and put her hand on his, "I'm sorry you had to go through what you did. I'd like to welcome you home. Thank you for your service to our country."

She said he broke out sobbing, stood up, and hugged her.

Everyone else in the waiting room started crying too. When the receptionist opened the door and saw everyone in tears, she asked, "What happened out here?"

"Another soldier was just brought home from Vietnam," Lorraine told her.

After she told me what had happened, Lorraine asked, "Can you imagine what would happen if everyone welcomed back just one veteran. Do you know how many souls might be healed?"

The Path from War to Peace: A Heroic Journey

Not everyone gets welcomed home by others, or even themselves. Guilt sometimes interferes with the process.

"Even some of the most grievously wounded Iraq-war veterans seem more disturbed by the killing they did than they are by their own injuries," Major Peter Kilner tells writer Dan Baum in an interview in the *New Yorker*.[5] A former West Point philosophy instructor, Kilner went to Iraq so he could write about the war's history. When he returned, he spent a week among amputees at Walter Reed Medical Center in Washington, D.C. "I was struck by how easily they could tell the stories of the horrible things that had happened to them. They could talk about having their arms or legs blown off in vivid detail, and even joke about it, but, as soon as the subject changed to the killing they'd done, a pall would settle over them."

"Pall" is a good word to describe soldiers' experience; I've seen it too. This pall is intended; it is a requirement for the battlefield. "To win war, the Army must turn soldiers momentarily, into reflexive, robotic killers," writes Baum. But there are consequences for these actions; Baum notes that during World War II, the American military lost more front-line soldiers to psychological collapse than to death by enemy fire. He quotes S.L.Marshall, a Lt. Colonel during World War I, who later became a reporter and quasi-historian of WWII: "Fear of killing, rather than fear of being killed, was the most common cause of battle failure in the individual." He cites Rachel McNair, who examined data from the Vietnam Vets Readjustment

Study for her doctoral dissertation: "Soldiers who had killed in combat (or believed they had) suffered higher rates of PTSD."

Baum also addresses the denial of governmental agencies to respond to the psychological distress that killing causes. Traditionally, he says, neither the Army nor the Department of Veterans Affairs surveys soldiers about the circumstances under which they killed, let alone how the incident affects them. For example, soldiers returning from combat in Iraq fill out a four-page form checking boxes that describe their experiences. The closest that the form comes to asking about killing is the question, "Were you engaged in direct combat where you discharged your weapon?"

Baum cites the VA's 207-page *Iraq War Clinician Guide.* He says it discusses the trauma of killing only with regard to civilian casualties, wholly ignoring the effects that killing enemy combatants might have. The Army's 500-page medical-corps text on combat trauma, *War Psychiatry,* is no better. It contains a chart that lists 20 "Combat Stress Factors," including fear of death, disrupted circadian rhythms, loss of a buddy, etc. The chart makes no mention of killing and offers no suggestions for ameliorating any psychological aftereffects, even though elsewhere, the text acknowledges "casualties that the soldier inflicted himself on enemy soldiers were usually described as the *most* stressful events."

A Vietnam veteran named, Dan Knox, is also interviewed by Baum. After serving two tours, Knox got married, had children, and held himself together while earning a law degree. But in 1995, one of his children died suddenly and his mental health deteriorated. Knox says that what bothers him most, more than 30 years later, is not the fear, not the carnage he witnessed, nor the loss of friends. It is the faces of the people he killed while serving as a helicopter gunner. "If they told me to kill a whole village, that's what I'd do," Knox says. "I still see images—a woman and her children rolling in the dust." When Baum asked Knox how often such images arise, Knox said, "Every 10 minutes." Later, he added, "Really, it's more like I'm always looking at a double image. I see you sitting there, and I'm also watching this funeral party I gunned. In a few minutes, it will be a sampan I gunned on a river, with a woman and her babies falling out of it into the water and kicking around as I shoot them."

Baum writes that on the day they were talking, *Time* magazine ran a story on Army snipers in Baghdad. A sniper who had killed seven men in one day was quoted as saying that he felt no remorse. "He's got the 'thousand-yard stare'," Knox replied tapping the photo. "Go back and find him in 15 years and see what he says."

Baum's report is not surprising to me. It explains why I see what I see as soldiers die decades later.

Paul was a patient who typifies the issues that Baum writes about. Paul was anxious and depressed when I first met him. He had received treatment for PTSD for many years. Now, he had liver cancer. The team gathered at his bedside for our usual QOL meeting and asked him if any of his experiences in Vietnam were still troubling him. Paul told us about two incidents that continued to cause him anguish. His unit had come upon a small village of huts that had been burned. Children were there without any adults. Paul felt certain that the younger children had subsequently died of starvation.

"I should have defied orders and carried out one child, maybe even two," he told us, throwing a pillow over each shoulder to show us how he would have done it. "I could have at least saved them." Paul's desire to help and protect native children is a sentiment I've heard many veterans express.

The other incident focused on his killing an enemy soldier who later proved to be unarmed. These two incidents haunted him. He remained stuck in the shame of his actions.

We listened to him without trying to take away his shame. Then we discussed the many symptoms he was experiencing, and spoke of options for treatment that could help him toward self-forgiveness. We told Paul we could design a therapeutic ritual where he could tell his story, seek forgiveness, and receive care and support to let go of his shame. "If it'll help, I'm all for it," Paul said.

We suggested that since he was Catholic, we could include the priest and he could go to confession during the ceremony. Paul agreed. His sister lived out of state and Paul wanted her to participate by phone.

We held the ceremony in the chapel. It opened with a prayer by Chaplain Dan acknowledging Paul's shame for his actions and his desire for forgiveness and peace. We then sang a song that reflected his need to separate from his old identity and past actions.[6]

Paul was then offered the opportunity to tell his story to the assembled group of five hospice and palliative care staff, the priest, and his sister (via speaker phone). He did this easily, repeating the story he'd told the hospice team.[7] Then Ed, one of the hospice volunteers who is a Vietnam veteran, drew in close to Paul and spoke about his own struggle with recovery from PTSD, highlighting similar feelings of guilt and shame. Readings from other Vietnam veterans that depicted their journey out of guilt and shame were then read. Paul's decision to say good-bye to guilt and shame was affirmed. We acknowledged he had punished himself long enough. A song of forgiveness, *Amazing Grace,* was sung. Paul and the priest then went to a nearby room for the sacrament of reconciliation while the rest of the team knelt in prayer.

When Paul returned to the room, we sang a song that conveyed new life, *Awake, Awake and Greet the New Dawn,*[8] and Chaplain Dan read the parable about the *Prodigal Son* from the Bible.[9]

Paul's sister was encouraged to participate. "I never knew Paul suffered so much," she said. "He never talked about his war experiences." She told Paul that she hoped he would now be free of guilt, free to enjoy life without its stain. She apologized for having never really known his pain, and expressed gratitude that he had opened himself so she could now understand him more.

Each team member then told Paul the impact his story had made on us and how inspiring his courage was. This was a very powerful time for Paul as he witnessed how he was making a difference in our lives. Guilt had bankrupted Paul's self-worth many years before. Letting him know he made a difference in our lives helped restore his sense of value.

A closing prayer acknowledged his release from past transgressions. Hope for a new future emerged. We then surrounded Paul with a group hug.

Throughout the service, Paul kept saying, "This means so much to me."

As we walked back to the Hospice and Palliative Care unit, Paul kept shaking his head in disbelief. "This touched my heart. It really did," he said. "It has moved me in ways I didn't know were possible. I feel I've been forgiven and I'll be okay now when I die. Thank goodness for all you in hospice for healing my heart."

The next morning while passing Paul in the hallway, he reached out and gave me a large bear-hug. "I want to thank you for yesterday, Deborah. I slept so well last night. I feel so good. I feel so free. I feel like . . . I feel like . . . ". He paused, then finally blurted out, "A virgin!"

I burst out laughing, not understanding his answer. "A virgin? What in the world do you mean Paul?"

"I feel so clean. I feel so pure. I don't even want to cuss. I haven't felt like this since I was a kid." It was wonderful to experience his childlike delight. Then with the same joyful expression, he added, "Can I die right now?"

I gasped and my knees became weak. Paul must have noticed. "No, you don't understand," he exclaimed. "I want to go out feeling like *this*."

All I could do was smile and hug him again. His request for death made me realize that the moral injury he had sustained had robbed him of much of his life, and he didn't want to risk it returning to rob him of a peaceful death.

Paul lived several weeks happy and free of symptoms. He had a new-found innocence; his delightfulness drew people into his presence. His sister flew in to enjoy Paul's new freedom and loving nature. She said the change was remarkable.

Sadly, the day before his death, Paul's anxiety and agitation returned. We treated his symptoms with medications, and he then died peacefully. I had to resist the urge to feel inadequate because his symptoms had returned. I knew that healing was seldom instantaneous or 100% complete, but rather an ongoing process.

Programs for Returning Soldiers from War

I fear readers might think I'm either promoting patriotism or that
I'm antiwar. I'm not sure I'm an advocate for either. As I've matured
from my idealistic "why can't everyone get along" attitude to acceptance of war as a human condition, I've accepted what I cannot
change. War has gone on for thousands of years and will no doubt
continue for thousands more.[10] I have simply opened myself to its
aftermath and tried to give that aftermath a voice. My hope is that
I've been able to convey a message that speaks not about me, but
about the needs these men and women have.

I do acknowledge that each Sunday when our church prays for
the protection and safety of our military, I add a silent prayer about
love and forgiveness for and by the enemy as well. I'm not sure if
that's aiding and abetting the enemy; I believe I'm doing what my
religion teaches me to do.

I have sometimes feared that acknowledging military service and
calling soldiers "heroes" might glorify war, thus blinding us to war's
realities. Now I realize that hope lies in our society's willingness to
help our soldiers recover from war and listen to the lessons they have
learned. When we are able to do that, we will then understand the
value of war recovery programs as much as we understand the value
of military induction programs. Because of what soldiers were
trained to do and the role assigned them by society, my hope is that
their need for reintegration into civilian life will be meaningfully
addressed. Just as the necessity for six weeks of "basic training"
indoctrinates soldiers into new military roles and identities, the
necessity for at least a few weeks of meaningful "basic civilian training" might help reintegration into a nonwarrior culture.
Homecoming ceremonies and cognitive reprogramming integration
exercises such as we used with Paul to "rehumanize" the "lean, mean,
fighting machines" (as well as their families) may help minimize
damage sometimes created by stoic walls. Just the fact that more
Vietnam veterans died of suicide after the war than died in the war
speaks of the perils that postwar soldiers encounter when they can-

not find peace.[11]

Programs to integrate combat trauma are especially important. The PTSD program at the West Haven Connecticut VA utilizes therapeutic ceremonies for combat-traumatized patients and their families.[12] The program relies heavily on Native American Indian purification rites for returning warriors. In one such rite, each discharged soldier goes on a long hike in which he or she is met by family and friends along the road welcoming him back. A ceremonial fire is lit, allowing each soldier and family member to release a burden that symbolizes the freeing of new energy and hope for the future. Each soldier plants two fir trees in the woods symbolizing the transformation of the wounded self through rebirth.

The West Haven VA also developed ceremonies for veterans entering and leaving a PTSD treatment program. Family members accompany a group of veterans for admission. An opening ceremony acknowledges the pain the veteran and their family have suffered, while expressing hope for recovery as the family releases the veteran into the treatment program.

A month later, families return for a ceremony midway through the program. They learn about the components of PTSD, including the fight/flight/freeze behaviors that often accompany it. The need to change abusive cycles and participate in the process of forgiveness is emphasized. Then participants are divided into groups according to their relationship with the veteran for the purpose of writing a collective letter to the veterans. All the parents join to write a collective letter, such as this one:

> Dear Sons and Daughters: We've experienced agony, anguish, anger, and fear for your very life when you went to war as well as since your return. We've seen you change from the happy wonderful child, proud to be in the service, into an angry withdrawn adult. We have lived with anger at the country, at the doctors, at the President. We did the best we could. We'd like to have you back.

We'd like to have your love. We love you. Your
Moms and Dads.

Spouses group together, composing a letter to the veterans such as:

Our Dear Spouses: You have made us feel hurt,
overwhelmed, alone, resentful, and empty. We
recognize you got the short end of the stick from
the government. We can't change that. We have to
make a fresh start and build for the future for us
and our children. The illness has consumed us
also. We miss the people we used to be. We want
you as our spouses and parents of our children.
We'd like you to open up. We want you as our
friend. Come home. Your spouses.

Children compose a collective letter that might read as this one did:

Dear Moms and Dads: We love you and we're
proud you are in the hospital getting help. We
think we know what your problems are but we're
nervous because we're afraid you might get mad if
we tell you. There are two sides to you. Sometimes
you're mean and destructive and sometimes you're
sweet and caring. Sometimes we want to hide the
keys to protect you from drinking and driving. We
see you making some success. We like it when
you're home to play with us. Love, your kids.

Veterans also write a collective letter, like this example:

Dear Family and Friends, We thank you for being
here, for standing by us after all that has happened. We know we haven't been the best example
as a spouse or parent or child. We are deeply sorry

for not showing enough love, for the abuse, for
not being sensitive enough to you, and not being
able to trust you. And for all this sacrifice, perhaps
you will get us back—willing to listen, with a new
attitude, and able to spend time with you and our
dear children. We look forward to the day when
we can look in your eyes and say "I love you" with
feeling . . . instead of harshness, tenderness . . .
instead of isolation, communication. We love you
so very much. The Vets.

After these readings, everyone rejoins their families, often with many
tears and hugs.[13,14,15]

Cemeteries, and Memorials: Healing Opportunities for Unresolved Grief

Veterans have much unresolved grief. On a battlefield, there's no
time or space to grieve. A comrade dies and grief must be numbed so
fighting can continue. Attention and energy are needed for survival;
grief is a distraction that could be fatal. It is important, however, for
the soldier to grieve as soon afterwards as possible. Otherwise, at
some point a friend or family member dies and the veteran can have
a disproportionate grief response. This exaggerated grief response is
good if the veteran uses it as an opportunity to go back and mourn
the deaths of his comrades. If he doesn't, he might become depressed
instead. Therapeutic rituals and ceremonies are one way to provide
healing forums for grief to surface so it can be transformed into
strength and wisdom. Military unit reunions can also provide healing. I've often heard stories about veterans not connecting with their
painful military past until attending a reunion where they received
strength and safety from their comrades in arms.

Memorials and cemeteries can also serve as catalysts for healing.
Our VA Medical Center has a national cemetery. A half-mile loop of
asphalt is edged with oak trees with Spanish moss gracefully swaying

from their boughs. The trees stand guard, providing quiet dignity for the veteran bodies reposed under their protection. I sometimes amble the eerie walkway. I pass cemetery markers, row after row, neatly arranged, precisely spaced, all stones the same, and all names and dates different. Some names I recognize, remembering their passing on the Hospice and Palliative Care unit; most names I don't.

Interspersed among the 25,000 markers are occasional visitors. Some bring flowers; some kneel quietly before graven images of memories still alive. Sporadically, there are small children whose parents are quietly teaching them the value of honoring the dead while instilling stories that will one day become their legacy.

On one of my walks, I see a man taking a lawn chair from the trunk of his Cadillac. I acknowledge his presence with a nod.

"You have someone here?" he queries.

I explain that I don't know anyone here personally. "But I've cared for many of these veterans before they died. I'm a nurse here," I tell him.

This excites him. "Let me show you the list of medications I'm on," he says happily, and shoves a list into my hand.

I scan two-pages of pharmacopia; most of these are for psychiatric conditions. "PTSD from World War II," he tells me. "I come here every day. My psychiatrist says it's good for me."

He explains that he had served in Japan as a medic. "We were targets you know." I hadn't realized this, so he explained that the enemy prided themselves in killing medics because they knew that meant many other soldiers would then die of their injuries. He said that injured soldiers couldn't even call out for a medic. "The Japs knew the word 'medic' and would call it out from the bushes to lure us over to them. Then we'd be ambushed."

We stood in silence while I opened myself to experience the gravity of what he had said. "Your comrades in arms are here. Even though they're dead, they're still your comrades," I finally comment.

"It's true," he says pensively, sweeping his gaze across the timbered lawn.

"I'm glad you have them. They understand you," I said, joining his studied survey of the surroundings.

The carillon strikes the quarter hour in its Big Ben style. On the hour will come 10 minutes of song. You never know what songs to expect. There are often military songs: *Anchors Away, Off We Go into the Wild Blue Yonder, Over Hill Over Dale.* Sometimes they are Beatles songs: *Here Comes the Sun, Hey Jude, Let it Be.* Today it plays pop: *New York, New York.*

My walks in the cemetery prompted me to attend a VA Memorial Day ceremony held there. It wasn't the Memorial Day speeches made by the Congressman or the General from a nearby Air Force base that impressed me that day, impressive though they were. What moved me was watching the hundreds of veterans respond to the speeches, the music, and each other. It was watching an elderly amputee struggle to get up during the National Anthem and the vet who came over to help him so he could stand at attention. It was the 25,000 small American flags flapping in the breeze, planted that morning on each grave by a local Boy Scout troop. It was watching two Gold Star mothers whose sons had died in Vietnam and Iraq, respectively, lead a procession to a monument.[16]

My sense of patriotism and pride was profound, yet I was aware of a rising sense of ambivalence. Do we use these ceremonies as a way of glorifying death so that families can feel that their loved one's war death was justified? Do we use this kind of pomp and circumstance to honor the dead as a way of military recruitment of those who may yearn for similar honor and glory? I didn't know the answers to those questions; I was simply aware of how these opposing sentiments could occupy the same space in my mind.

My ambivalent wonderment about war and peace continued. A few months later, the Medical Center's employee recreation and service organization sponsored a drive to collect Christmas presents for soldiers in Afghanistan and Iraq. A list of needed items had been provided. It included candy, games, CDs, crosswords, and batteries. It also included Beanie Babies for the soldiers to give to village children. With the help of our hospice and palliative care social worker, Karen, whose husband Jaron Jones was stationed in Baghdad, we set up a wrapping and packaging center in my garage. She would then mail all the boxes to her husband for distribution to his comrades.

I invited my 8-year-old granddaughter, Ashyln, to participate in our enterprise. She arrived with 10 Beanie Babies. I was surprised and moved; she had been diligently collecting the Beanie Babies each time she went to McDonalds to eat. She was very protective of them; no one could play with them, including herself. She was waiting until she had the complete collection. I was pleased with her generosity and her reason for giving. "They need them more than I do, Nana," she told me.

Nothing could prepare me for the e-mail forwarded from Karen's husband, however. It was from a comrade in Fallujah:

> Yesterday we were in a convoy of about six armored humvees when suddenly the first humvee stopped. There was a young girl sitting near the middle of the road, and she would not move no way and no how. The commander of the unit gave the order to be nice to her and just go around her. As I passed the little girl, I recognized something in her hand. I radioed for everyone to stop and went over and knelt in front of her. I recognized her and the Beanie Baby I'd given her a few days earlier. I tried to get her to move off the road. She shook her head "No." Then, she pointed right behind her back. I bent over to look and there it was . . . a large land mine big enough to destroy one of our armored humvees. This little girl was doing her best to protect us from running over the mine. Because of this, you won't read in today's news: "A roadside bomb exploded as a US military convoy went by." Abu Musab al-Zarqawi and some of the other adults we are now fighting were once children. I wonder what life would be like over here if we had given them a beanie baby when they were children?

Lessons Learned

- Veterans' identities can persist long after discharge from military service.
- "Thank you for serving our country" is a small thing to say, but it can make a big impact. It requires sincerity, however; words become trite and perfunctory when they don't come from personal exploration and development of awareness of the sacrifices veterans have made.
- Acknowledge families of veterans. They, too, have often been through hardships, especially if the veteran had PTSD or if the veteran had made a career of the military, which required frequent family moves and transitions.
- It's never too late to say, "I'm sorry."
- Whether we win a war or not, whether a war is just or unjust, does not change what soldiers went through, the sacrifices they made. In fact, losing wars or fighting in wars they come to believe are unjust make the sacrifices that much more difficult to bear.
- Rituals can be an important, often overlooked, format for precipitating healing because they access the unconscious. Effective rituals incorporate three stages: separation, transition, and integration (Appendix E).
- Military reunion events, military cemeteries, and war memorials sometimes act as catalysts to precipitate healing by bringing experiences out of the darkness into the light so that peace can ensue.
- "Abu Musab al-Zarqawi and some of the other adults we are now fighting were once children. I wonder what life would be like over here if we had given them a beanie baby when they were children?"

Chapter Six

Farewell to Arms: Coming to Peace

Hoping and wishing
you can settle
this whole thing in your mind
about this war
resolving it within yourself
before the time of atonement comes
weeping and crying at the end of your life.
—*Atoning* by Ron Mann[1]

A VA Hospice can serve as a place for wartime *at-one-ment;* it's one last chance to become at-one with unpeaceful memories and to reckon with the guilt of deeds inhumanly committed during human wars. I have sometimes seen memories surface with "weeping and crying at the end of life," as veterans deal with the moral residue of war. I've learned that the at-one-ment process begins by acknowledging guilt that veterans sometimes harbor. Some feel guilty about killing. This moral injury they sustain can sometimes haunt them if they haven't reckoned with it previously. Others feel guilty for *not* killing. More than one veteran has told me that they shot a man and couldn't do it again. "They had to take me off the front lines. I was such a coward." Some even feel guilty when they sustain an injury that does not allow them to remain in combat. "All I could think about was leaving my comrades behind."

Noncombat veterans sometimes feel guilty when fellow soldiers volunteer for dangerous missions. One of my patients was a talented trumpeter who was assigned to the Navy band, playing as ships left harbor for Vietnam. Tearfully, he told me, "Here I was with this cushy job playing an instrument I loved to play. It wasn't fair."

Another veteran told me the trauma he vicariously sustained with his job handling body bags. "Each of these guys could have been me, except that I was here counting their corpses." I've even seen combat guilt in a man who was never a soldier at all. He was sitting at his father's side on our Hospice and Palliative Care unit. The son told us how he had been a conscientious objector during the Vietnam War. Later, he became a psychologist and found himself working with Vietnam veterans. "I have a lot of guilt about the impact my actions had on them."

I've heard stories of guilt from nurses and medics about the life and death decisions they made. One veteran told me she wasn't afraid of hell because "I've already been there. I have to live every day with the faces of those soldiers who didn't have a chance during mass casualties. The doctor left it up to me, a 21-year-old nurse, to decide which ones got surgery and which ones were left to die."

Survivor's guilt is common. It can interfere with veterans' ability to enjoy their lives. One World War II veteran told me, "When I landed on the beach, there were all these dead bodies. The sand underneath them was pink with their blood." Then he tearfully added, "They didn't get to have grandkids the way I did. It's not fair that I should have this enjoyment when they can't."

The *at-one-ment* process often begins by forgiving others, including those on the other side—the "enemy." Many have been able to do that early in their civilian lives; others harbor hatred that continues to poison their vitality. Some Vietnam veterans struggle with forgiving the government for using and betraying them. Korean and Vietnam veterans might have to forgive the American public for ignoring or scorning them. Forgiveness isn't just between people either. Soldiers have to forgive the world for being unfair and for having cruelty and war in it; they have to forgive God for allowing the world to be like it is.

It is the inability to forgive one's self for letting others die or, worse, for killing others that keep some veterans in darkness; shame seals light from their souls. It is this moral injury that soldiers sustained that I sometimes see surface as they lie in a hospice bed facing their own deaths. Experiencing or witnessing violence can be disturbing for anyone; but the difference with veterans is that they *committed* much of the violence. That is a deeper level of traumatization. Such was the case with James.

James was weak with a cancer that would take his life in a few days. After I introduced myself and we spoke quietly for several minutes about hospice care, I asked him what he needed so he could have a peaceful death. He said he had something to say but he was too ashamed to say it out loud. Motioning me down to his pillow, he whispered: "Do you have any idea how many men I've killed?" I shook my head, remaining silent, steadily meeting his gaze with my own. He continued. "Do you have any idea how many throats I've slit?"

Again I shook my head. The image was grim, and I felt my eyes begin to tear. James was tearful too. We sat silently together and shared his suffering. No words need be said. This was a sacred moment that words would only corrupt.

After several minutes, I asked, "Would it be meaningful if I said a prayer asking for forgiveness?"

He nodded. I placed my hand on his chest, anchoring his flighty, anxious energy with the security of my relaxed palm.[2] My prayer, like any praying I do with patients, reflected no particular religion. "Dear God: This man comes before you acknowledging the pain he has caused others. He has killed; he has maimed. He hurts with the pain of knowing he did this. He hurts with the pain of humanity. He comes before you now asking for forgiveness. He needs your mercy to restore his integrity. He comes before you saying 'forgive me for the wrongs I have committed.' Dear God, help him feel your saving grace. Restore this man to wholeness so he can come home to you soon. Amen."

James kept his eyes closed for a moment, tears streaming down from beyond unopened lids. Then he opened his eyes and smiled gratefully; his new sense of peace was almost palpable. It was a reminder to me of just how heavy guilt weighs.

This sort of guilt is not unusual among combat veterans. Some loved the rush of the killing and later have guilt for having enjoyed it. One veteran who had been an especially effective sniper during the Korean War, tearfully lamented his pride in his expertise. "I won many awards for marksmanship, but now I can't believe how much pride I took in being able to pick them off. That's what hurts the most." He reminded me that though snipers can be a long way off from their victims, the killing is very graphic because the scope magnifies the target. Others have guilt for killing women and children. Killing enemy soldiers can at least be justified; civilians' deaths cannot, nor can the accidental killing of comrades in what is called "friendly fire." I have also heard stories about the intentional killing of officers who consistently made poor judgments that jeopardized lives of those they commanded.

It's tempting to try to soothe the guilt away with rationalizations: "That was a long time ago" or "You were just obeying orders." Rationalizations don't help, however. They know when and why they killed, and whether or not it violates their deepest-held moral beliefs. What they need is to have the guilt acknowledged and accepted so that finally they can forgive themselves.

If self-forgiveness seems like a lot to expect, it is; but it's also essential. To withhold forgiveness means to cut oneself off from a compelling force deep in the soul that seeks it. If that forgiving force is denied, vitality and peace remain elusive. If someone is unable to achieve forgiveness, they might arrive at the end of life filled with bitterness. Stockpiling transgressions of others (blame) or self (guilt) is the recipe for making bitterness. Bitterness is a poison that contaminates even the most innocent heart.

Memorial monuments, such as the Vietnam Wall in Washington, D.C. can be a catalyst for healing bitterness. Monuments often serve as a repository for shame, precipitating the courage to seek forgiveness, such as a photo of a North Vietnamese soldier with his daughter left at the Wall. It was left by the soldier who killed him with the following note attached:

Dear Sir, for 22 years I have carried your picture

in my wallet. I was only 18 years old that day we
faced one another . . . Why you didn't take my life
I'll never know. You stared at me so long, armed
with your AK-47, and yet you did not fire. Forgive
me for taking your life. So many times over the
years I have stared at your picture and your daughter, I suspect. Each time my heart and guts would
burn with the pain of guilt. . . . Forgive me, Sir.

Later, this soldier went to Vietnam to meet the little girl in the photo
personally so he could ask for forgiveness.[3]

I can only imagine that beyond the guilt this man felt was a
heart that yearned for peace. In fact, sometimes I think that war and
peace are inversely related. The ravages of war sometimes cause its
participants to crave peace and kindness. I asked a sister of one of our
patients how the Korean War had changed her brother. "It made him
kinder," she said. "He came back much more concerned about other

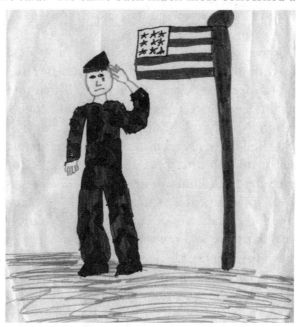

"The Price of Freedom" by Ashlyn Grassman, age 11

peoples' feelings. He was never like that before the war." Another combat veteran told me that he had studied to be an engineer before he had gone to war. "But afterward, I decided to become a doctor. I wanted to make up for the things I had done in the war. I wanted to help others."

War: Forgiveness Issues on the Other Side

Veterans are often tasked with forgiving the enemies they were fighting if they are to experience life without bitterness; their enemies are tasked with the same. The D-Day Museum in New Orleans has many video clips of veterans among its exhibits. One clip shows a Japanese pilot who had bombed Pearl Harbor. He speaks about how badly he felt for being part of the sneak attack. Such attacks, he says, go against his samurai code; attacks were supposed to be out in the open so they could be fair.

In the next scene we see this pilot meeting with one of the Pearl Harbor survivors. They talk about forgiveness. The Japanese veteran leaves a rose at the Pearl Harbor memorial to honor the soldiers, sailors, and marines he had killed, acknowledging his remorse. Now he sends the American veteran money to leave a rose at the memorial annually.

Forgiveness issues also surround those who are not combatants on either side. The natives of the land where warfare takes place are often traumatized or left with their lives drastically altered. Occasionally soldiers marry natives of the places where they were stationed, and I get a glimpse of war's effects on the people of the land where wars were fought. However, it was a Hungarian patient named Matthew who taught me most about the effect of war on those who, unlike Americans, experience war on their own soil. Matthew came to the end of his life filled with wisdom that was mixed with bitterness. His bitterness was born from wartime experiences he had endured when he was a child. Listening to his story, I realized how wartime forgiveness is needed not only by our veterans, but by natives and enemies alike. When there is violence, forgiveness is needed by all involved.

I had asked Matthew to fill out a Life Review form. The Life Review form asks questions that promote reflection so meaning about the value of a person's life can be acknowledged. It helps people realize that their life has made a difference and has not been lived in vain.

I sometimes compile the reflections from the Life Review form into a ritual for the patient and family, like having the funeral before the patient dies, so he can participate. The public telling of the patient's story provides witness to the significance of their life. Matthew agreed to such a ritual.[4] I gathered his story over several sittings. He was too weak to speak any length of time. He completed it the same way he faced his dying; there was no evidence of feeling while intellectualizing his experience. The complexity of his story also demanded careful attention and consumed energy that sometimes was beyond his reserve. When he grew fatigued, his Hungarian accent became more difficult to understand. Still, he persevered. "It's important," he'd tell me.

I also mailed Life Review forms to Matthew's two sons to complete before the ceremony; they flew in for the event. The ceremony began with the songs, prayers, and Bible verses that Matthew had selected. I then read Matthew's story. It showed us war from the perspective of one who had experienced it first hand, not as a soldier but as a civilian in an invaded country.

"You were born in 1932 in Gyor Hungary," I began. Then I spoke about how Matthew's happy early childhood had been shattered by World War II. Threatened by both Germany and Communist Russia, Hungary became an increasingly difficult place to live, and in 1944, he and his family fled the country along with hundreds of other refugees. They got as far as Austria where they became officially "displaced persons" living under military rules with no legal status. "You were not even recognized as refugees. The United Nations had various programs for Displaced Persons, DPs as you came to be officially called. International law should have prevailed, but it seldom did. You were classified as 'stateless'."

The family was finally able to immigrate to America. "You said that what stands out most about your childhood is your struggle for life and self-preservation." The struggle for life didn't stop after Matthew reached American soil. Six months after arriving, his father suddenly died. "The responsibility of caring for your family now fell on your 18-year-old shoulders." This family responsibility was able to help Matthew maintain a deferment for a few years, but at age 24 Matthew was drafted into the Army for the Korean War. He was bitter about this.

I added my own response to his reaction. "I was surprised when you told me this. I thought you would be grateful to the country that had given you refuge, but I had not known war. War was all you knew, and it was the last thing you wanted to participate in, whether as its childhood victim, its teenage refugee, or as a young adult soldier. You had just survived a lifetime of wartime conflict, and now you had to go into another. It didn't seem fair, but fairness usually is not an issue in war." Matthew served two years in the army in Korea reconstructing bridges, even winning medals for doing so. "It must have felt strange to be rebuilding a war-torn countryside that was not your own country—displaced yet again."

When Matthew was discharged from service, he used the GI bill to gain a degree in International Trade and Finance. He embarked upon a distinguished career that included over 20 years of executive management in the field of domestic and international trade and finance. His personal life, however, was chaotic and difficult, always reflecting the fear and insecurities of his early years. After he retired, Matthew joined some investors in Florida to form an aircraft leasing company. "Unfortunately, the investors were fraudulent and you lost all your assets. These last few years have found you 'displaced' yet again."

The ceremony closed with some insight from Matthew. "The thing you like best about yourself is that you are an 'honest, straight-forward' man. Coming to the end of your life, you leave one piece of advice: 'Stay true to yourself. Stand by your values and beliefs'." This part was followed by some of the responses on the Life Review forms his sons had completed. "Doug remembers an intense struggle over custody. He appreciates that once the divorce was settled, he and his brother were never 'used as pawns' between you and their mother. Aaron says that when he thinks about you, he thinks of how 'fiercely independent' you are. He also thinks of how 'stubborn' and 'private' you are, adding that talking about you is like talking about himself because you two share many qualities. He says he loves you and will miss you."[5]

After the tribute, Matthew's sons thanked us. They had known little of their father's early life. "My father could be a stubborn SOB who had to control everything," Aaron said ruefully. Now that he understood how little control Matthew had as a child in a war-torn land, he could appreciate his need to control his circumstances as an adult. Understanding brought congruence to what had appeared to be an incongruent life.

Matthew lived a few weeks longer. He liked the mural that the staff had painted on the wall showing a road with footprints marking patients' journeys. I asked Matthew what these footprints meant to him. "They mean 'Together we walk, one step at a time'," he said slowly and precisely. We added his words to the top of the mural.

A few weeks later, Matthew lay dying. A blooming narcissus sat on the windowsill, yielding its beauty as the sun rose on the horizon beyond it. "Look Dad. It's springtime," Aaron said, belying the December day that it was. "You love flowers," he said as he plucked them for his Dad.

Matthew clutched them tightly, crying. He died with the flowers in hand.

The Aftermath of War: A Time of Atonement

Matthew had lived under the specter of war his entire life. Understandably, he still harbored resentment about war's effect on him. He had never previously considered forgiveness as a pathway to the peace he sought. I believe forgiveness is essential because it brings peace with the past. Though it is true that we cannot change the past, we can change *our relationship* to the past, and forgiveness is the means whereby we do that.

One crucial component of self-forgiveness is learning to distinguish guilt from shame. Guilt is natural and designed to provide feedback so we can learn important lessons; shame is artificially created and designed to punish. Guilt tells us something we did is wrong, guiding us toward more compassionate actions of others; shame tells us that we are wrong, consuming our self-compassion. Guilt mobilizes us into new behaviors; shame can immobilize us so that we remain stuck. Veterans with PTSD are often filled with shame. They need to go from shame to guilt before they can get to forgiveness.

I've also learned the importance of identifying "false forgiveness," those times when a patient says, "I let that go a long time ago" or "It's over and forgotten." Sometimes, that's the case. Other times it's a way to fool themselves so they can sidestep the work of forgiveness. I know, because I'm guilty of practicing false forgiveness myself.

Sometimes people resist doing the work of forgiveness because they think it will then condone what was done to them. "What happened is still wrong," I tell them. "And until you achieve forgiveness, that act—as awful as it is—is still controlling you."

I also explain how forgiveness is a process that often has to be done incrementally over time. "It doesn't just happen," I caution, snapping my fingers. I explain how the process starts with wanting to forgive; this step is the most crucial and also the one most vulnerable to omission due to self-deception. People say they want to forgive, but their actions often belie the stated motive. If the patient has a spiritual orientation, I often simply ask them to start the process by praying for a *willingness* to forgive. If spirituality has no meaning or if the word "forgive" has an unwanted religious connotation for the patient, I usually speak in terms of holding onto something versus letting it go. Often I provide a simple homework assignment of having them write down: "I want to forgive _____" (myself, name of someone, a situation, etc.). They tape this to a mirror and say it each day. It's amazing how powerful this simple exercise can be.

Sometimes, we explore the purpose nonforgiveness serves and the role it may be playing in sabotaging forgiveness efforts. This role might include receiving sympathy for the victim role or staying safely stuck in powerlessness so no risk is taken to assume responsibility for their needs or to ask for their needs to be met.[6]

Asking people to consider forgiveness without pressuring them is important. Because I've seen peace come to people when they do the work of forgiveness, I've developed a bias toward wanting everyone to do it. I have to resist imposing my bias on others, remembering that people may not be able, ready, or willing to forgive. I not only need to accept this, I need to understand and respect it. My job is to encourage them to consider doing the work of forgiveness, but I have to be careful that I do not judge them if they choose not to. When I don't completely respect their decision, small inflections in my voice or changes in my posture give me away; the patient experiences my judgmental attitude and withdraws. When this happens, opportunities to help them consider forgiveness at some future time are lost. This is a significant loss. Not unusually, I open the door to forgiveness and the patient declines to enter. This doesn't mean that they don't want to forgive, it often means that they are not yet ready. When I initially see patients to discuss forgiveness, they might not be interested. As death approaches, however, I often remind them about the possibility of forgiveness and, not unusually, they are then ready, willing, and able to forgive.[7]

It's also important not to rush people into forgiveness prematurely. "Forgiveness should not come until guilt has moved us into remorse. Remorse is realizing how our action hurt others," I heard a presenter at a hospice conference say.[8] "Otherwise, forgiveness is just a self-indulgent, guilt-relieving device that does not lead toward compassion." He's right; I've seen that too.

Physician M. Scott Peck writes about guilt in a similar way. In his book, *The Road Less Traveled*,[9] he identifies a "disorders of responsibility" spectrum. On one end of the spectrum are people who don't assume enough responsibility for hurtful actions. When there's conflict in their relationships, it's the other person's fault. Relieving them of guilt without exploring it so they can develop a sense of remorse means the gift of guilt is missed. To tell such people, "You were doing the best you could" or "It's not your fault" only reinforces their reluctance to accept responsibility. Instead, guiding people toward realizing the impact of their actions on others can birth compassion, generating apology and forgiveness. For example, we were having a QOL meeting with Peter, a patient in our community living center. His health was failing, and he was scared he might die. When we explored this, he revealed that he used to belong to a motorcycle gang. "I watched lots of women get gang-raped," he told us.

I was struck by Peter's lack of emotion. I asked him about the effect this had on the women. He didn't know, remaining more focused on his guilt than on their pain. There seemed to be little remorse, so he was unable to elaborate. When we closed the meeting, the patient requested a hope for the day. When my turn came, I fought to abide in my nonjudgmental self so I could sincerely appeal to a sense of compassion that Peter seemed to lack. The fact that he told us what he had done suggested he might be ready to take responsibility for it. He couldn't feel the pain of what he'd done, but if I stayed open and connected to him, maybe I could feel his pain for him so he could feel it for himself. With emotion, I offered, "My hope for you this day is that you reflect on what you did to the women you watched get raped so you can understand the pain you caused by witnessing their harm without stopping it. My hope is you will let yourself feel the pain of those women . . . not for their sakes, but for your own so you can sincerely feel remorse and ask for forgiveness." I then offered that at some point he could think about doing something especially nice for a woman in his life so that those raped womens' suffering will not have been in vain.

Peter looked me in the eyes, gave me a slight nod of his head, and said, "Thank you."

Unlike Peter who assumed too little responsibility, some people assume too much. They are on the other end of Peck's disorders of responsibility spectrum. When there is conflict in their world, they not only shoulder their own guilt, but everyone else's. When something goes wrong, they assume they're at fault. They drown in remorse, or more accurately "false remorse," taking on guilt that isn't theirs. They need encouragement to let go of inappropriate guilt. This was the case with Ed. You may remember Ed from Chapter 4. He was the Vietnam veteran who volunteers on our Hospice and Palliative Care unit "so no more veterans will be left behind." Ed was visibly upset when he asked to speak with me. "I've been sitting with Mr. Bailey. The phone rang, and I went out to answer it and when I came back, he had died." Just talking about what had happened escalated Ed's anxiety.

"Are you saying you knew he was going to die in that few minutes that you stepped away and so you said to yourself, 'Oh Goodie, here's my opportunity to let this man die alone?'" I asked.

"No. I didn't know he was going to die right then."

"Good. For a minute there, I was starting to think that you thought you were God and that you were omniscient and could have predicted the moment Mr. Bailey was going to die."

Ed laughed. "No. I don't want to be God."

"Then are you willing to forgive yourself for being human and not being able to predict the future?"

Ed said he was. We also talked about whether his exaggerated guilt response could be a remnant of a lack of self-forgiveness for the comrade he had left behind years before.

"I don't think so," Ed said thoughtfully. "When I wrote that letter, I really was able to forgive myself." Ed said he thought the patient's death was simply a trigger for his PTSD which caused the memory of his comrade's death to surface.

"That's an important distinction you're making," I responded. "In that case, open up to the memory. Tell your comrade hello and remind him that he still lives on in the work you're doing here helping other vets. Thank him for coming."

Ed smiled and expressed relief.

Helping people like Ed develop an appropriate relationship with guilt is like separating wheat from chaff, sorting out what to hold onto, what to let go, what is realistic and what is unrealistic, what is their business and what is not. As Peck says, "What we are and what we are not responsible for in this life is one of the greatest problems of human existence. It is never completely solved. It requires continual assessment and reassessment."[10] Peck's observation reminds me of the famous Serenity Prayer: "God grant me serenity to accept the things I cannot change, courage to change the things I can, and wisdom to know the difference."[11]

I've come to appreciate how peace and forgiveness are inextricably intertwined, even in small ordinary ways. I have to forgive every disappointment and interruption that interferes with my experience of the moment. To be at peace, I have to forgive the world for things not going the way I had hoped; then I can reencounter the ever-present now; I reestablish atonement in my world.

I've also come to realize that forgiveness may be the simplest and hardest thing each of us are asked to do; to not forgive, may be the most foolish because we might arrive at the end of our lives filled with bitterness. Bitterness is a venom for the soul.

I suspect that Rachel Naomi Remen shares this belief. In her book, *My Grandfather's Blessing*, Dr. Remen tells a story about a well-known rabbi who was asked to speak at a Yom Kippur service on the topic of forgiveness. Yom Kippur is the Day of Atonement when Jews reflect on the year just past, repent their shortcomings, and hope for God's forgiveness. The rabbi went into the congregation carrying his one-year-old daughter. The little girl smiled at the congregation, then she patted her daddy's cheek. He smiled and began a traditional Yom Kippur sermon. Feeling his loss of attention, the baby grabbed his nose. He freed himself while he continued the sermon. Then she took his tie and put it in her mouth. The congregation laughed. The rabbi retrieved his tie, but the little girl grabbed him around the neck. Looking out over her head, he told the congregation: "Think about it. Is there anything she can do that you could not forgive her for?" Just then, she grabbed his glasses. Everyone roared. After settling his glasses back on his face, he asked, "And when does that stop? When does it get hard to forgive? At age three? At seven? At fourteen? At thirty-five? How old does someone have to be before you forget that everyone is a child of God?"[12]

Transforming from Killer to Child of God

I have often seen how veterans with PTSD live in isolation. I had
assumed it was only to protect themselves from having to deal with
others; but as often as not, I've found that isolation is for the sake of
others. They sometimes sacrifice their own hopes of having families
because of the suffering they fear they would cause other people.
George was one of these. He was a quiet man who had lived with his
mother most of his life, caring for her as she grew old and frail. Now,
she visited him as he lay dying on our Hospice and Palliative Care
unit. I sometimes wondered why this nice man had never married. I
found out one day when I asked him about his war experiences. He
looked at me for a moment, sighed deeply, and said, "I was with
Lieutenant Calley."

I must have looked stunned because he added dryly, "I can see
you know what that means."

Yes, I knew. Vividly the headlines came back to me. My-Lai.
The massacre of innocent villagers. The story had polarized the
nation. I remembered the country's confusion and division over
court-marshaling a man performing an ill-defined wartime job.

I nodded. "Yes, I know what it means. It means you've either
lived with a lifetime of guilt for killing those people or a lifetime of
anger for being accused of doing it."

"It was the guilt," he said. "Years and years of guilt. Guilt I can't
describe because when I looked back on what happened, I couldn't
believe what we'd done." For years, he'd tried to erase it from his
mind, eventually realizing that he had to face it, accept his guilt, and
do whatever he could to atone. "It took me years of running from it
and then working on it before I could come to peace with it."
Meanwhile, his mother knew what he had done and helped him deal
with his anguish. "She kept praying for me. Never judging me. Never
pushing me." He began going to church and this helped, but My-Lai
still tormented him. By the time he felt confident that he'd made

peace with what he'd done, he was 45 years old. "I had always want-ed to get married, but I had already been a burden to my mother. I didn't want to take a chance on being a burden to a wife. I couldn't be sure the torment wouldn't come back. I had to accept that I was-n't fit to have a family." His mother was getting older. She had stood by him through all his suffering; he decided to devote his life to hers. "I had hurt enough people. I had the chance to help one person. I wasn't going to let it pass by."

It was hard to see in this tired, peaceful man, the monstrous killer he had once been briefly. He had accepted his guilt, and with-out self-pity, he had made the atonement that he could. I realized he had given me the chance to see what redemption really meant.

Forgiveness Doesn't Always Relate to Military Issues

More typically, guilt that arises at the end of life surrounds issues that occur as part of everyday living, as these next two stories depict. Phil had been in World War II, but he had not suffered PTSD. His health was failing and the past few years had become frustrating, taking its toll on his relationship with his daughter Carol.

"He has to have everything just right," Carol told me. "He yells whenever things don't go his way. I hate to see his life end with our relationship like this," she said ruefully.

I asked Carol about her father's childhood as well as his military experience, searching for clues to what was causing his lack of peace and his escalation of distrust. Carol said she knew little about his childhood, and all she knew about his military career was that he had served in World War II. So I met with Phil to ascertain these things directly. As he told me his history, I had little trouble understanding why he tried to keep his world ordered, controlled, and rule-driven.

"I never told Carol about my childhood because I'm ashamed of it," Phil said hesitantly when I met with him. "You see, my father was the town drunk." Phil had been laughed at and humiliated. "I'll never forget my mother looking up one day and seeing a horse eat-ing grass on the side of the road and saying, 'Look. Someone at the bar must have strapped your Dad on the horse and sent him back in our direction.' Of course, Mom would bring him in and wait until his drunkenness wore off and life would go on." There was also a lot of violence. "Mom won the physical assaults because Dad didn't fight back. I guess he thought he deserved it," Phil said forlornly. "I'm not sure what he told the doctors when he was hospitalized with the broken ribs and bones; I'm sure it wasn't the truth because everyone covered up for each other. One thing I know. There was no love in our home growing up."

I felt sad just listening to Phil. At age 75, the pain still stabbed Phil's heart. "Later, it was cars instead of horses. I can't tell you how many times we would find Dad's car pulled over to the side of a road with him laying half in and half out." Through it all, his mother covered up for him, beat his dad up, and left Phil and his brother unprotected and without any sense of emotional security. "All the activities and awards I got at school, my Dad never knew about. Actually, he didn't even know if I was in school or not. All he knew was how to get his next drink and how to make it home after his last drink and how to endure my mother's verbal and physical assaults in between."

When he got older, Phil's relationship with his father remained based on hurt and shame. "One of my worst memories was when my bosses took me out to a restaurant to tell me they were promoting me. It was a great time of celebration and I was on top of the world," he said lighting up with the memory. "When we came out of the restaurant, there was a large crowd gathered in the street with the police. To my shocked dismay, there Dad was, stone drunk in the middle of the street. I didn't know what to do. If I said anything, my bosses would know." But Phil told the policeman it was his father and he'd take him home. "The policeman had already called the black Mariah to take Dad to jail. So I stood by helplessly and watched as they slung my father, unconscious, into the back of the truck like a piece of meat. The indignity of it hurt all the way through me. Of course, my mother bailed him out, and it all started over again."

Phil said his military years were difficult too. He tried not to think about them. "I really can't describe how lonely military life is. One day you're a young man in familiar surroundings, and the next, you're plucked up with hundreds of other soldiers and you don't know a one of them. You find yourself overseas where nothing is familiar in the midst of a war, a war that has given me a lifetime of memories I've tried to shut out and run from as best I could. No man should see some of the things I've seen." He paused a long time before resuming. He said the only time he wasn't scared was the week he went on pass in France. "Anybody who says they aren't scared when bullets are hitting all around you and shells are coming down upon you, is lying." He said he was also afraid of friendly fire. "Some of the new guys were trigger-happy, and they weren't afraid to shoot at anything that moved. It's hard to see your buddies shot up because a new guy was too scared to see who they were shooting."

His role in the war was to run telephone wires. One of the jobs that scared him the most was when his tanks got tangled up in wire and he was sent in to take care of it. "I figured that the enemy knew the tank was there and that someone would be sent to retrieve it so I was an easy target. Each time I approached, I really did expect death. Even if I escaped that, what greeted me was almost as bad. Sometimes it was the soldiers shot. Sometimes they were stabbed. You just can't believe what humans can do to each other," he said haltingly, his voice cracking with emotion. "I was only a boy myself. It really made me sick. Still does. But I don't want to get my mind in some of these places." Then he added proudly, "Meanwhile, we kept the wires up. A lot depended on that!"

The military taught him self-control. "Growing up, I had little self-control. For years after I got out, family members commented how much I had changed because I had learned self-control." He said learning self-control was good but "war changes you in ways that can't be described. Maybe a few ways are good. Many are bad. And probably most are not even known."

I asked Phil about how his experiences had shaped his relationship with Carol. "As I grew up, I knew one thing for sure: I would never put my kids through what I had been through," he said. "I made a decision not to drink or smoke. I would not bring shame to the family name. I would hold a steady job. I would be successful. My children would be proud of their father. They would never have to know the humiliation of neighbors and strangers laughing at the town drunk. They would never have to wonder where Dad was." He was proud that he was a self-made man. "I rose against the odds and I made it. God's been good to me. He made up for the childhood I had."

We talked at length about how he had covered up his shame with success. He said he felt certain that the way to achieve success was through strict self-control. As we spoke, he realized how his fear of shame ended up controlling him. He began to see how this had imprisoned him in a rigid lifestyle that constrained his relationships. Once he realized this, he had little trouble seeing the effect this had on his daughter.

Quickly he agreed to write a letter to his daughter so he could leave a different legacy than the one he had begun. He started the letter by telling his daughter the details of his history. Then he provided Carol his new perspective:

> I didn't want pain and shame to touch my own family. Unfortunately, it did anyway. It just wore a different mask of shame and hurt. I like most about myself those things I liked least about my father. As a little kid, it's so scary to not know where your Dad is, if he will show up, what he will look like when he's found or even if he will be alive, or what rampage your mother will go on that will land your Dad in the hospital or jail. My brother and I only had each other to cling to helplessly while we watched and silently cried out for it to stop. I thought if I worked hard enough and became successful enough, my children would be proud of their father. I thought that would be the best gift I could ever give. Now, I realize working

long hours at work and renting the farm and being with the horses all the time left you alone and feeling forgotten. I thought I was making people happy. Neighbors were proud of us. You kids didn't have to hang your head in shame every time you walked down the street. You didn't have to be laughed at when you walked by someone. There was laughter and no loneliness. I thought that was love. You see, when I was a child, I don't ever remember laughter in my house. I don't ever remember a house without loneliness. I don't even remember a house that anyone visited.

You are helping me see that this was not such a gift after all. My preoccupation with making you proud of me meant you didn't see me much. I didn't realize that was important. I liked it when my Dad wasn't home. It may have been lonely but it was quiet. I thought as long as I was out working hard, staying busy, being responsible, and bringing honor to our name, I was being a good father. It never really dawned on me until now that you suffered my neglect. It never really dawned on me how much it hurt you to be ignored because of my need to make you proud of me. It never really dawned on me until now how much I didn't pay attention to how different you are than me. I didn't see you as a little girl with your own thoughts and feelings. I assumed your needs were the same as mine had been when I was a kid. I still have trouble with that. I still want to tell you how to think and feel because I forget you are your own person. I realize now how self-centered that is. I thought I was giving you the father you always wanted. Now I realize I was giving you the father *I* always wanted and I cheated you out of the father you needed.

I'm ashamed of the verbal attacks I've had with you over the past few years. I don't believe you deserved that. My pride and my thinking you should think like me made me blind to what I was doing. I ask your forgiveness for that now.

Carol, I love you. I showed love in the best way I knew how: to work hard, be responsible, be punctual, be honorable, maintain my senses and control, all so you would feel proud and not suffer embarrassment and humiliation. I'm so sorry this left you ignored and abandoned. I'm so sorry it has meant that I didn't see you as your own person and assumed you would want for yourself what I wanted for you which was really what I had longed for as a child for me. I'm sorry I cheated you out of the Dad you needed me to be because I was too blind to find out what that was.

I'm ready to die. Waiting. Glad for it. I say that out of joy. Joy for my Maker and his Son. In recent years, I have tried to live my life as a good Christian as best I can. I still have many potholes, but if you look for the potholes, you'll always see them. I know that God forgives me for the potholes I've created. He's filled them up with love and peace and He doesn't even see them. I'm ready to be with Him. My only hope is that you can forgive me for the ways in which I have let you down. Certainly, the last thing I ever wanted was to hurt or disappoint you or make you not feel proud to have me as your father. Please forgive me. Dad

When Phil gave the letter to Carol, she was tearful and understanding. "It's okay. You don't need to apologize," she said to him. I often do what Carol did: I rebuff the gift of apology and forgiveness that someone offers rather than receiving it openly. I do this because I think it spares the apologizer's feelings by letting him off the hook. Unfortunately, it often does just the opposite; it misses the opportunity to receive the apology and affirm the value of the apologizer's intentions. Now I recognize the value in giving them the satisfaction of my opening their gift and receiving it graciously with, "Thank you. That means a lot."

Carol was extremely grateful for the insights her father provided her. The letter provided explanations that filled in unknown gaps. "I knew Dad's childhood had been bad, but I didn't know how bad it was. I'd always assumed it was me, that I was unlovable. Now, I realize it had nothing to do with me. The funny thing is I realize now how much he did love me. He was trying to protect me from experiencing what he had experienced. That was love and I just didn't know it."

I was also grateful for Phil's insights. I told him how his courage, honesty, and humility were teaching me things I needed in my own life. He seemed pleased, adding yet another bit of wisdom. "Learning is what I take with me when I die," he said with a twinkle in his eye. "What I have taught others is what I leave behind."

Fight, Flight, Freeze: Instincts to Avoid Confronting Feelings and Memories

The man in this next story had a similar abusive past as Phil; however, rather than fleeing into perfectionism, he had fled into drugs. The journey he made in order to accomplish forgiveness, however, was no less courageous. With a lifetime of unfinished business from chemically coping with life rather than reckoning with its difficulties, Darryl was a tough character. Alcohol and drugs had been self-soothing substances that sabotaged his ability to heal the brokenness in his life, which led to his getting AIDS. The HIV team asked me to intervene.

"He's going to die in a few weeks if he doesn't get dialysis," the nurse told me. "But he doesn't want it. All he wants is his drugs." She explained that he had been in the substance abuse program and failed it several times and so he was no longer eligible for treatment there.

When Darryl came into Hospice and Palliative Care clinic for an admission interview a few days later, he looked sick because he had many blood abnormalities that dulled his mental capacities. He said he was willing to stop his cocaine and start dialysis. He must have seen that I looked surprised because he added, "I've tried and messed up before. But yesterday I went to my cousin's funeral. When I looked into the coffin, I told myself, 'Next time that will be you in there'." He said it really shook him up.

"I'm sure you were shaken before and you've said you were going to quit hundreds of other times too," I said skeptically. "So, what's different about this time? You haven't convinced me this is going to be any different."

Darryl explained that he had had a dream in which God had told him to reform his life. He also said his mother was weary of drugs, guns, and broken promises. The previous week, she had called the police when she found a stash of drugs and guns in an abandoned car in the yard.

"Good for her!" I told him, watching for his reaction. "That's just what she should do to help you."

Darryl also had a son. "Is your drinking and drugging a source of pain and embarrassment for him too?" I gently asked. Darryl acknowledged it was. "How would your life be different if your son were proud of you instead of embarrassed?" I asked.

Darryl had no difficulty painting a vision of changed relationship with his son and the new meaning this would provide. He also wanted to reach out to his cousin's young sons. With their father dead, they needed guidance. I realized this could be another potential source for him to discover meaning in his life.

"If I decide to accept you for our hospice program, we'll have a big investment in you. What assurance do we have you won't betray us the way you've betrayed yourself and your family through the years?" I said. "Convince me this time is different."

Darryl could provide no assurance, a sign he was becoming more honest with less flighting into denial and illusions. He seemed sincere, and there was an important difference in his current situation. He had been doubly humbled by God and by death. He would need both to expand into the spiritual dimension so his life could be transformed.

The next day, I met with the general medicine and HIV teams, along with Darryl and his mother. His mother remained skeptical and guarded, but she was also prayerful and hopeful. I commended her endurance, her continued support of her son even after he'd proven untrustworthy, and her wisdom in calling the police. She cried with the validation of her suffering. "At my age, I can't keep it up much longer though. I'm hoping this is the answer to my prayers," she said.

Because Darryl could die in the next few weeks if he didn't receive dialysis and because he was no longer eligible to receive treatment for his drug abuse, we admitted him to the Hospice and Palliative Care unit so we could provide an emotionally safe environment with imposed protection from drugs. Recalling Darryl's determination not to be in a coffin, I placed him in a room with an imminently dying patient, hoping it would provide reinforcement for his motivation to avoid drugs. The patient, Mr. Brown, had a similar history to Darryl's. Released from prison for terminal care, Mr. Brown had appeared to be imminently dying for weeks. With no family in the area, the team speculated that he was waiting for someone, some friend or minister or family member, to come so he could die.

On Darryl's first night, Mr. Brown struggled. Darryl came to his bedside and comforted him, holding his hand and praying. The next morning, the team gathered at Darryl's bedside for a QOL meeting. Darryl told us what had happened with Mr. Brown; we smiled at each other. Though Darryl had been put there to gain benefit from Mr. Brown's death, Mr. Brown had also benefited from Darryl.

Just then, Mr. Brown's breathing slowed. The team rolled our chairs from Darryl's bedside to form a circle around Mr. Brown. We invited Darryl to join us, affirming how his care had helped Mr.

Brown. "We think he was waiting for someone who understood and accepted him. You were that 'family' for him, Darryl," I said. At that moment, Mr. Brown took his last breath.

I recruited Darryl into further work, telling him I would continue to give him roommates who needed his care. I also explained boundary setting and encouraged him to speak his need and let us know if the responsibility was beyond his ability or his needs.

Darryl was learning new coping skills distinct from his past fight, flight, or freeze addiction reactions. He realized it was going to be a difficult change. "Fightin' is alls I knows," he explained in his thick African-American dialect. "It's what I learned on the street growing up. It's what the army taught me so I could save my life. I have to be 'da man' (with macho gesture) or I die." Suspicion and lack of trust in others were necessary for survival. Stoic walls had, indeed, probably saved his life.

Darryl then added another source of his suffering. Darryl's drug contact, "Easy Money," had recruited him into storing drugs. Darryl had kept the stash in the couch cushions. Not realizing the stash the couch contained, his wife bought a new couch, giving the old one away. Darryl got irate, an action which recently precipitated divorce. "I's never hurt so much," he told the team. "Help hold me up 'cuz I knows I can't."

Sometimes Darryl still acted anxious and suspicious. It was difficult to know if his behaviors were related to drug withdrawal, personal coping mechanisms for dealing with death, or ingestion of more drugs. I asked for an order for a drug screen. Darryl felt betrayed.

"I tole yous I'm not gonna use drugs nomo. Why won't yous believe me?"

"Look Darryl," I said sitting down low before him, staring him squarely in the eye and placing my hand on his shoulder. "I want to believe you. You want me to believe you. The drug test will help that happen." His history, I reminded him, made it impossible for us to fully trust him, or for him to even trust himself. If his drug screen came back negative, that would increase our willingness to stick with him. If it came back positive for drugs, then we'd have to discharge him home.

I expected resistance or at least an argument, but Darryl relaxed, even giving a half-smile. "Yeah. I gets that. The drug test is gonna show yous that yous can trust me."

"There's nothing that would please me more Darryl," I said sincerely, acutely aware he would be doomed to a despairing death if the drug screen came back positive. Thankfully, the results of the drug screen proved negative. Darryl gloated his victory. I enjoyed that too.

A few weeks later at a Memorial Day bereavement program in which people were sharing their stories of loss, Darryl took the microphone and explained he had AIDS from drug abuse. He told the crowd that more than anything, he needed to learn how to trust "and it starts with surrounding myself with people I's can trust. I've decided to stop fightin' yous folks and let yous help me." The crowd responded with applause. He confirmed his intention by adding, "This is the first time I've ever *voluntarily* told anyone I have AIDS."

Darryl had learned the value of revealing himself to trustworthy people and being accepted so that he could stop fighting and instead ask for help. He was doing the work of healing, building a trustworthy world where he could feel safe enough to come out from behind walls that had kept him a "fightin' man."

During subsequent QOL meetings, Darryl often prayed. His prayers were simple, humble, and sincere. His mother was usually present. At one meeting, he rose from his bed, got on his knees before his mother and asked for forgiveness. It was a powerful moment for Darryl; it began his process of replacing manipulation with reckoning. For his mother, it symbolized the culmination of years of fervent prayer for her wayward son. For the team, it was the marvel of being privileged witnesses. I never felt as proud of anyone as I did at that moment with Darryl.

Darryl was discharged home, returning to the Medical Center for dialysis three times each week. Though it was difficult, he remained clean and sober. He cared for his mother. He had gotten actively involved with his cousin's children. He visited the Hospice and Palliative Care unit for the weekly breakfast the chaplain, physician, and volunteers provided, sharing his success story. He credited his transformation to the power of God.

"You offer hope to your son and cousin's sons," I told Darryl. "If they ever get in trouble or get mixed up in drugs, they'll remember it's never too late to make a different decision and turn their lives around."

"Yeah. Yous right. Theys already tole me theys proud of me."

Two years later, his body weakened with complications, Darryl returned to the unit for hospice care. His mother tended him tenderly and gratefully. "He'll be going home soon," she told me. "We're going to have a big home-going ceremony for him next week," she explained.

"Home-going ceremony?" I queried.

She laughed with my lack of understanding. "In our culture, this world ain't our home."

"Ah. I've got ya," I laughed with understanding. "It's been a long way back home for Darryl," I noted.

"You got that right," his mother responded. "But his home-going is going to be so different because of what happened in these last two years," she smiled.

I could only nod with satisfaction. Darryl had worked hard these past two years. He had role-modeled the humility, courage, and honesty I needed to seek in my own life. He had become the hero in his life the way I wanted to become in my own.

Lessons that Bring *At-one-ment*

- Combat veterans sometimes feel guilty or ashamed about the killing they did. This moral injury they sustain can sometimes haunt them if they haven't reckoned with it previously.
- Some veterans feel guilty for *not* killing. Some have to forgive comrades for unjustifiable acts that the veteran felt powerless to confront. Noncombat veterans sometimes feel guilty when they have seen fellow soldiers volunteer for dangerous missions. Nurses and medics may feel guilty about the life and death decisions they made. Survivor's guilt is common; it can interfere with veterans' ability to enjoy their lives. Others have guilt for killing women and children, committing "friendly fire," or the intentional killing of officers who consistently made poor judgments that jeopardized lives of those they commanded.
- Depending on the war, there are many people and institutions to forgive, including the "enemy," the government, the American public, the world, God, and most importantly, themselves.
- Don't try to rationalize away guilt with, "That was a long time ago" or "You were just obeying orders." Instead, recognize that they are seeking forgiveness.
- It's important to assess where someone is on Peck's disorders of responsibility spectrum that ranges from no guilt to irrational guilt. We need to respond differently depending on which end of the spectrum the veteran is on.
- Forgiveness may be the simplest and hardest thing each of us are asked to do; to *not* forgive, may be the most foolish.
- Forgiveness is needed not only by our veterans, but by natives and enemies alike.
- If a calm person places their hand on an un-calm person's sternum, it can often help them feel secure, more weighted, less anxious.
- If someone is unable to achieve forgiveness, they might arrive at the end of life filled with bitterness.

- *Wanting* to forgive is an essential, often forgotten, element of forgiveness. Affirmation or prayer can help achieve this.
- Respect the decision a person makes about whether or not to forgive.
- If someone is unable, unwilling, or not ready to forgive, patiently wait for another opportunity and ask them to reconsider it. However, be careful that they do not experience any pressure or judgment.
- Memorial monuments can be a catalyst for healing bitterness.
- Though it is true that we cannot change the past, we can change our relationship to the past, and forgiveness is the means whereby we do that.
- A crucial component of self-forgiveness is learning to distinguish guilt from shame.
- Beware of "false forgiveness," those times when a patient says "I let that go a long time ago" or "It's over and forgotten."
- Don't rush people into forgiveness prematurely.
- Don't rebuff apologies with, "It's okay. You don't need to apologize." Instead, receive the apology openly.
- "War changes you in ways that can't be described. Maybe a few ways are good. Many are bad. And probably most are not even known."
- "Learning is what I take with me when I die; what I have taught others is what I leave behind."
- Let others inspire you with humility, courage, and honesty so you can become a hero in your own life. Then peace can reign.
- Interventions can facilitate the forgiveness process. (See Appendix B)

Chapter Seven

Myths, Metaphors, and Symbols: The Language of the Unconscious

The heroes of all time have gone before us.
The labyrinth is thoroughly known.
We have only to follow the thread of the hero path,
and where we had thought to find an abomination, we shall find a god.
And where we had thought to slay another, we shall slay ourselves.
Where we had thought to travel outward,
we will come to the center of our own existence.
And where we had thought to be alone, we will be with all the world.[1]
—Joseph Campbell

Most of us have certain images of military "heroes." These images often reinforce stoic facades that remain undaunted by interior or exterior circumstances. Many people contend that any person who has served in the military is a hero. For myself, I don't apply the term unilaterally. Just because someone joined the military or fought in a war or survived an injury does not automatically qualify them for heroic status. All have done things they are proud of; all have done things they are ashamed of. Some performed heroic deeds in the military, but failed to apply courage in living their personal lives. Other soldiers suffered crippling emotional experiences in the military and applied learned lessons to their personal lives; these are the heroes who have inspired me.

In his book, *The Power of Myth*, Joseph Campbell writes about the kind of heroes about whom I speak. He says that myths show us how we can each be a hero in our own lives. "All the myths deal with transformations of consciousness of one kind or another. You have been thinking one way, you now have to think a different way."[2] He says this occurs either by trials or illuminating revelations. It is the hero who learns to respond to trials by gradually awakening deeper dimensions within.

Most of the heroes in my life have been patients like Mr. Elliott. He had lived a troubled life after World War II. While many might hail him a hero because of what he endured while in a German prisoner-of-war camp, I found him heroic because of the courage, honesty, and humility with which he lived his life after the war. Suffering from terrifying flashbacks and consumed with maintaining control, he had lived with the ravages of PTSD. I met Mr. Elliott when Hurricane Charlie was threatening the coast of Florida, forcing evacuations of low-lying areas. Arrangements were made for him to be evacuated to our VA Hospice and Palliative Care unit. His turmoil and suspiciousness were evident upon arrival.

"Now that I'm here, I guess you're going to lock the gates so I can't escape," he said when I greeted him.

I assured him that the gates were not locked, that he was free to leave at anytime, and that our only intention was to keep him safe during the hurricane. He received little comfort from my words. His agitation continued while we worked to get his anxiety and paranoia under control.

"You all seem nice on the outside," he said, "but I know it's just a matter of time before I find out that you're all Hitlers on the inside."

"It's okay," I responded. "We'll let your wife keep you safe. She can give you your medications; she will protect you from any Hitlers." We had his wife sleep at his side, give his medications, and broker all cares that were needed.

"I can only take a shower, no bathtubs," he said. Then he explained that the POW guards had dug a hole and put him into the ground to interrogate him. "They left me there for hours. I had no control. They determined when I would get out."

I told him there'd be no confinements for him, including bathtubs.

After a few days of repeatedly reaching out to him, providing antipsychotic medications, and creating a safe loving environment, Mr. Elliott calmed down and began responding to our efforts. As we've often experienced with our veterans, he even became tender. Mr. Elliott's end-stage heart disease limited his survival to just a few weeks; he wanted to go home to die. After the hurricane had passed, we made arrangements for him to return home with home hospice. As he was leaving, we asked him if he wanted a prayer to send him on his way. He did.

"What do you want us to pray for?" Chaplain Dan said.

As is often the case, the hero perspective emerged. "I want to pray for all of you. I came here thinking you all were going to execute me and came away realizing that you're my salvation." He then prayed for each of us and our families. Even though we had seen this kind of graciousness with hundreds of other veterans, our team looked at each other in amazement. All that he had suffered during the war, all that he had suffered with his PTSD after the war, all that he was facing in the next few weeks, and he remained focused on us. Then he added the hero perspective that helped us understand why. "People need you. People out there are struggling . . . people in all their imprisonments trying to get out."

Heroes Are Willing to Struggle out of Their Imprisonments

Awakening deeper dimensions so we can be free of inner imprisonments is no easy deed. It requires courage, honesty, and humility to recover from the effects of trauma by using the experience to grow and change. I frequently use the words courage, honesty, and humility throughout this book; I do so consciously because they capture the qualities I believe we each need to cultivate if we are going to be heroes in our own lives. It takes courage to let go of our fears and instead show up for things in our life we'd prefer to fight, flight, or freeze. It requires honesty to let go of illusions, denials, and pretenses so that we can open up to our authentic self, including the aspects of ourselves we'd prefer to hide. Paradoxically, humility empowers us; we gain real power when we let go of pride and will power and open up to acknowledge our needs and ask for help.

I see these heroic qualities every day as I care for patients like Mr. Elliott. As they are dying, chaos all around them, they express gratitude. They die with grateful hearts.[3] I've come to appreciate how desperately our death-denying American society needs role models for how to die healed. These veterans can show us. Combat has changed them in fundamental ways that shape, mold, destroy, and redeem the rest of their lives. In one aspect of their lives or another, they're able to redeem portions of their suffering so it can be used for healing. The process doesn't happen automatically; it's often an arduous journey. Their sufferings are often redeemed with wisdoms beyond earthly knowledge.

It was a story in Clarissa Pinkola Estes' book, *Women Who Run with the Wolves,* that completely changed how I understood and responded to combat veterans. One of her stories addresses people with PTSD and the anger that can accompany trauma: "Rage corrodes our trust that anything good can occur. Something has happened to hope. Behind the loss of hope is usually anger; behind anger, pain."[4] I recognized the truth of her description about PTSD. I had seen the rage and pain that the aftereffects of trauma sometimes caused. I had seen how bitterness sometimes squeezed life from war-torn souls until they became shells, hardened and lifeless, dead in bodies that are alive.

Estes, a Jungian psychologist, demonstrated a totally different approach to PTSD through the mythological story, *The Crescent Moon Bear.*[5] In this tale, a warrior husband returns from war behaving distantly and cruelly toward his loving wife. The wife turns to the village healer for help. The healer tells her she must find the Crescent Moon Bear who lives at the top of the mountain and bring back a single hair from its throat.

The trip to the mountain is perilous. The wife has to overcome numerous obstacles, but finally she finds the bear and feeds it every day until it is used to her and trusts her. She is rewarded by obtain-

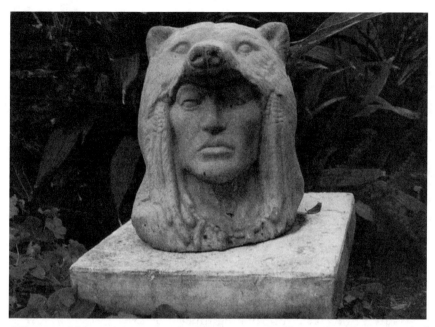

*My personal "Crescent Moon Bear," a gift for my garden from a friend, Pat McGuire.[6]
It gives me courage for my own journey of integrating scattered pieces of broken self into
a peaceful whole.*

ing the hair and returning to give it to the healer. The healer takes it, nods and smiles, and then throws it into the fire where it is instantly consumed.

"No!" cries the young wife in horror. "What have you done!?"

"Be calm. It is good. All is well," says the healer. "Remember each step you took to climb the mountain? Remember each step you took to capture the trust of the Crescent Moon Bear? Remember what you saw, what you heard, and what you felt?"

"Yes," said the woman, "I remember very well."

The old healer smiles, and says, "Now, go home with your new understandings and proceed in the same ways with your husband."

"En-couraging" Others to Meet their Crescent Moon Bears

This story helped me realize the difficulty families have in greeting and welcoming back their soldiers. Yet, author Estes emphasizes that the story is not about loving someone with PTSD. She says the story is really about the journey of emotional healing made by the person *with* PTSD. After the physical self comes home, the emotional self has to come home, and that can be an arduous journey.

Each character in the story actually represents different aspects of the self: husband (angry and tormented self); wife (loving self); healer (wise, calming, healing self); bear ("great compassionate self"). Estes says the story depicts what must be done "in order to restore order in the psyche, thereby healing the angry self:"

- Seek help from a wise, calming, healing, inner force (going to the healer within)
- Accept the challenge of going into mental and emotional territory not approached before (climbing the inner mountain)
- Recognize illusions that make you want to fight, flight, or freeze (obstacles threatening inner growth)
- Solicit the great compassionate self (patiently feeding the inner bear and receiving its kindness)
- Understand the roaring side of the compassionate self (recognizing that the inner bear, the compassionate self, is not tame).

Estes says the story demonstrates our desire to have something (a hair from the bear) or someone (healer) magically erase trauma. Instead, healing comes when we come down off the mountain and apply the lessons learned from having reckoned with our trauma.

The myth resonated with my own experience with suffering. For many years, I had avoided, denied, or reacted against the suffering in my life. I now realized that what I had been doing was avoiding making the trek to meet my Crescent Moon Bear. Instead, I had tried to get people who caused me suffering to meet *their* Bear, so I wouldn't have to meet mine. I read *about* suffering and how to transcend it, hoping my knowledge would magically make my suffering disappear. I had been willing to do anything *except* set foot on the path to meet my Crescent Moon Bear; I had lots of excuses why I didn't need to meet that Bear. After reading about the Crescent Moon Bear, I realized that it wasn't until I had suspected my Bear had something I needed that I was able to gather the courage to embark on the arduous journey to meet her. Paradoxically, I discovered that joy began to be slowly birthed into my life.[6]

"You can always tell those patients who've met their Crescent Moon Bear," I told our team one day. "Those who have, know how to abide and reckon with walled-off pieces of self and integrate suffering instead of run from it. They have a peace beyond worldly understanding." I realized that those patients had been my teachers and were still helping me in my mission of helping warriors come home from war so they could experience peace. The Crescent Moon Bear story now gave me a compass to guide my actions more deliberately. Now I saw my role as helping veterans climb the mountain to meet their Crescent Moon Bear. Death is one last opportunity to meet that growling Bear of Compassion and discover the gifts within. This meant patiently, humbly, honestly, and courageously abiding with their anger, pain, guilt, and helplessness so they could discover their compassionate self. It also meant helping them resist the urge to look outside themselves for a magic hair or healer.

The process reminds me of a story Karina, an art therapist, told me. She had suggested to a combat veteran that he paint his feelings about his war experiences. He painted a corpse. He became upset and said he wouldn't explain its meaning nor would he paint any more. Later, he asked for some paint-by-number art supplies, which Karina provided. He subsequently became obsessed with filling page after page with the numbered shapes. He plastered his walls with his prolific output. When I heard this story, its metaphorical significance impacted me. It depicts the aftermath of war on soldiers; their souls are no longer creations of art but rather furtive attempts to keep compartmentalized pieces together in some semblance of a meaningful whole.

Retrieving these fragments of scattered, hidden selves is the task after trauma, and it helps precipitate a peaceful death. Now that I had a graphic context to guide my interventions, I decided to be more deliberate in my response to war trauma that I encountered at the end of life. A patient named Sam Peters provided the opportunity.

My acquaintance with him began with a call from his home hospice nurse who was desperately requesting an inpatient hospice admission for him. "You've got to admit this veteran. He can't get any rest. He thinks there are Vietcong under his bed. None of the medications we are giving are helping."

"Tell him we can help," I responded. "Tell him we'll have a mattress on the floor for him so no one can hide under his bed."

Quickly I let the rest of the staff know to expect a "hospice code," that is, a developing situation that requires intensive response. Like code blues when a patient's heart stops and staff respond with CPR (cardiopulmonary resuscitation) to get the heart and lungs started, hospice codes get the veteran's emotional heart beating and create a sense of safety so the emotional lungs will trust the world enough to breathe it again. It's not easy. These kinds of situations are fraught with danger but they're also ripe for opportunity. It often requires unconventional tactics like those of the healer in *The Crescent Moon Bear*. It always requires being trustworthy.

The patient arrived agitated and wild-eyed. Like many Vietnam vets, he distrusted the federal government, and that included the VA and anyone who worked for it.

"Hi Mr. Peters. I'm glad you're here. I think we can help you," I said with tentative confidence, looking him gently and squarely in the eyes. I avoided calling him by his first name.

"Yeah? How ya gonna do that?" he responded suspiciously.

"I don't know yet. I don't know you. My job is to listen. You'll let me know."

"You've got the bed on the floor," he said both matter-of-factly and inquiringly.

"Your nurse at home told me you had trouble with Vietcong under the bed. The Vietcong may not know you're here, but just in case, I put the mattress on the floor."

"Uh huh," he grunted, checking out the room warily. I waited patiently, giving him space and time. Swooping in and taking control would only make him feel confined and cause him to want to fight or flight.

"You know. I really don't want to be here," he finally continued.

"Okay," I said. "As soon as you feel better, we'll get you back home."

Mr. Peters just looked at me uncertainly.

"Would you like a beer?" I offered. I had forgotten to ask the home hospice nurse if alcohol was important to him, but I knew vets often used it to numb painful intrusive memories, part of the "flighting" process. We kept beer on hand in case it was needed.

He looked at me incredulously. Half-laughingly, he rebutted, "No one's offered that to me when I've come to this place before. They're always telling me to *stop* drinking."

I explained that the Hospice unit had different rules from the rest of the hospital. He wasn't in hospice for rehab; rather, he was approaching the end of his life. We wanted to help improve the quality of his remaining time. Beer might help to do that. "If it's whiskey, I can get that too, but it'll take a little longer because I have to have the pharmacist bring it."

Still looking unbelieving, Mr. Peters said he could use a beer. "But make it a cold one. Warm beer . . . there's nothing worse than warm beer," he added.

I left, grateful for the struggles our team had previously engaged in about letting patients use alcohol on the unit. It had taken years for us to realize that if patients were dying at home, they would have access to their alcohol. Not only that, desperately needed hospice care was often refused by patients who were dependent on alcohol because they needed the comfort of the bottle and did not want to go through painful withdrawal. We reckoned with our personal objections and collaborated with hospital administration to provide physician-ordered, pharmacy-dispensed, nurse-administered alcohol.

I returned with an unopened beer and handed it to him. I watched as he popped the lid, regarded the spit of foam rising over the top, and sighed with satisfaction before taking a long gulp and then placing it on the bedside table. I began to talk with him. We'd deal with admission forms in a little while, but for now it was important to create a personal bond between us.

"You've had a hard time of it," I said, validating the suffering I knew he had probably experienced.

"Yeah, well . . . " He said no more.

I waited quietly with him until he seemed open to talking. "What's been the hardest struggle for you?" I finally asked casually so he would feel no pressure to respond. For years, my fear of causing harm kept me from pushing or prodding. "Don't go there unless the patient asks you to" was a safe motto to follow. It took me a long time to realize the problem was not "going there." The problem was my not knowing *how* to go there. Once I realized this, I realized the harm I was doing by *not* going there, not opening the door to their suffering. Not opening the door meant I abandoned them to the agitation and isolation they sometimes experienced at the end of their lives. Agitation and isolation is not a death I want to sentence anyone to.

After a moment, Mr. Peters spoke. "The hardest thing is closing my eyes," he murmured. "Whenever I close my eyes, I see faces . . . " his voice trailed off.

I waited again and then gently prodded. "Could you tell me a little bit about what the faces look like?"

"Blood. Bloody . . . and mad . . . sort of mad and sad at the same time. They start out looking like Vietcong, but sometimes they turn into demons. I just want them to go away."

He looked at me challengingly. I knew this look. It was a test to see if I could really listen without judgment. Then he added, "You probably think I'm crazy . . . "

"No. Not at all," I said. I assured him that many of the vets I'd worked with had horrible nightmares and even visions about the war. He needed to know that others had experienced what he had, that he was not alone, and that he was neither weak nor crazy.

He nodded but looked away, not wanting me to see his fear. He has learned his stoicism well. I leaned in closely, and noting that he didn't pull back, I touched his knee. These vets need the comfort of human touch, but they're often afraid of it. I talked about the courage it takes to acknowledge fear. Tears welled up in his eyes. He brushed them away, shaking his head as if in disgust.

"Tears are welcome here," I told him. "They're part of the healing process. We say that the only bad tears are uncried tears. It's good to see you release them."

Slowly he nodded. I lowered my head and eyes to give him emotional privacy.

Finally, I ventured further. "Can you tell me more about the people you see when you close your eyes? What do you think they want?"

He took another sip of his beer. His voice was shaking. "I don't know . . . I think they just want to scare me as much as I scared them."

"So, these are people you've met before? Maybe killed in combat?"

He nodded.

"And they've come back to do to you what you did to them? To kill you the way you killed them?"

He nodded, and I asked him to close his eyes and tell me what he saw. When he hesitated, I reassured him that he wouldn't be alone with the demons and that I was there with him to help.

Mr. Peters relaxed back on his pillow, closing his eyes tightly. After a moment, he haltingly reported the images he was seeing, symbolic images alive with guilt. "I see his face and the whole side of his face is gone. I see all the blood."

"What would you like to say to him?" I asked.

He didn't say anything for a long while. Then haltingly he started to answer. "I'm so sorry I did that to you . . . " Then a rush of tears burst forth and he began to sob. I waited. After the tears passed, I asked him what it was that he had done.

"I need to get out of here," he said suddenly, opening his eyes wide and searching the room for the exit. I realized I'd moved too quickly.

"It's okay," I told him. "You can leave if you need to. See if you can try breathing. Deep breathing. Tell the soldier to wait while you breathe." I breathed deeply with him. His "flighting" eased. "Mr. Peters, I'm sorry. I shouldn't have asked you that. You don't need to tell me what you did." I suggested that he tell the man in his vision what he had done to him. "You can say it silently; I don't have to hear. On the other hand, if you'd prefer to speak out loud, it won't upset me. There's probably nothing you can say I haven't heard from other combat veterans."

Mr. Peters closed his eyes again. He began to mumble to the man. After a time, he opened his eyes and was silent.

"What do you hope for him now?" I ask gently.

"I just want him to be at peace. I don't want him to have to wear all that blood. I want him to have his face back."

"Tell him he's welcome here and that he need not be afraid. Ask him if he will let you clean off the blood. Ask him if you could help him restore his face. Imagine a new face, a peaceful face." On we go . . . carefully . . . slowly . . . breathing . . . crying . . . couraging.

"Would you be willing to ask him to forgive you for doing what you had to do?" I resumed. "Maybe ask him to forgive you for hurting him, for killing him, for all the things you've done to all the Vietcong and any others during that war . . . "

Quickly and earnestly Mr. Peters did so. He lay there quietly. Finally, I asked him what he was experiencing. "I don't know. His face is back, but he's not leaving."

"Maybe he needs your forgiveness too," I said in wonderment. Mr. Peters opened his eyes, startled. "He's done things to you too you know." Knowingness slowly crept into Mr. Peter's face and he closed his eyes again. After a few moments he said the man was leaving. "He's sort of smiling. I've never seen him look like that before."

"Wish him well and bid him peace. Tell him you don't hate him anymore and that if he comes back, to come bearing peace and you will bear peace for him. You're both peace-bearing soldiers now."

"Yeah. We can make a truce," he said. Mr. Peters seemed peaceful for awhile, but then became tense. "Do you think they'll come back or are they gone now?" he asked, searching for reassurance I could not give.

"I don't know. They might. If they do, it's all right. You know how to talk to them now," I told him. He still seemed skeptical. "If the faces come back," I continued, "that's a good thing. It lets you know there's still work to be done. Just welcome them and ask them what they want. If you can't come to truce, tell them to come back later. Then, you and I can talk again and you can get back with them."

Mr. Peters seemed satisfied with the plan. He no longer had to "fight, flight, or freeze." He had a means to integrate traumatic energy.

The next day, Mr. Peters asked for his mattress to be put back on the bed. The Vietcong were gone. I marveled at the difference a day could make. I used to think I was too busy for these kinds of dialogues with patients. Now, I realized that having these dialogues actually gave me more time. Without them, I would have used valuable resources to provide one-on-one nursing care. I would have spent time listening to staff who worried about how to respond to his unmet needs while feeling frustrated trying to care for other patients who also needed their attention. I would have wasted time and money medicating what cannot be medicated. No amount of morphine can take care of this kind of pain. In fact, medication sometimes complicates trauma. Medication does not necessarily help these veterans feel safe, which is, ultimately, the aim of all interventions in these kinds of crises.[7]

For Mr. Peters, encountering the figures diminished their hold on him. Though the images later returned, he had developed a dialogue to confront the images; they become less menacing, and he felt more empowered. Not talking about the images only gives them power, and the veteran remains alone and terrified.

Though these kinds of situations do not commonly arise, when they do, we need to know how to respond. There have been times when I hadn't recognized the look that hides the torment, or I recognized it but hadn't known what to do, or I knew what to do but had been afraid to do it. The look of war is bone-chilling. We need to know how to see the look and how to respond to it. We tell our patients that they have to face their fears; we, too, have to face our fears if we are to be any use to them.[8]

Metaphors: The Language of the Dying

Soon after my work with Mr. Peters, a new staff member joined our team. Isla had been caring for her dying mother at home for two months. She said her mother had become confused, talking about a train that was in her room.

I wasn't sure it was confusion. "When people are dying, their conscious mind recedes and their unconscious mind expands," I explained. "The language of the unconscious is symbols and images. Transportation, travel, or 'going-home' metaphors are very common as people are dying. You'll see it in our veterans. They often speak in battle metaphors."

"Oh my gosh. I've been telling Mama there *is no* train," she groaned.

We talked about questions she could ask that would help her determine her mother's needs. That evening when her mother again spoke about the train, Isla listened carefully and intermittently asked questions.

"Where's the train going Mama? Who's on the train? When's the train leaving?" Most importantly, "What do you need to get on the train, Mama?"

"I need you to get on with me," Mama said in response to the last question.

Isla was stunned at first, not knowing how to respond; but then she answered calmly, "This is *your* train, Mama. You go ahead and get on it. I'll catch another train and meet up with you later . . . "

Her mother seemed satisfied, relaxing peacefully. Having received her daughter's blessing, Mama boarded the train the next day. Isla felt grieved, but she also felt at peace knowing she had contributed to her mother's peaceful dying.

I was glad I'd been able to help Isla. I hadn't always been so familiar with the use of metaphor with the dying. Just as *The Crescent Moon Bear* had opened my eyes to the value of mythological stories in healing trauma, the book, *Final Gifts,*[9] opened my eyes to the role of metaphor in the dying process. Written by two hospice nurses, it awakened my conscious mind to the power of the unconscious. I began to study the language of the unconscious.

I wasn't unfamiliar with symbols, images, and metaphor. After all, each night when my conscious mind slept, my unconscious became awake with dreams. Like a magician who makes audiences think rabbits can disappear, my conscious mind often invisibilized information derived from the unconscious by forgetting dreams, ignoring their meaning, or discounting their value. Now, I began to notice that during the dying process, as people are letting go of the outside world and transitioning into an inward one, they begin speaking the language of the unconscious. The invisible rabbit is now pulled out of the hat—this time for all to see and hear, if they have eyes and ears that have learned to value rabbits.

It was the study of metaphor that led me to the writings of mythologist Joseph Campbell. I also began to read the works of psychiatrist Carl Jung. These authors helped me understand the value and power of symbols to access the healing energy of the unconscious. Symbols speak what words cannot, awakening us to dimensions words can't reach. Symbols touch the larger self.

Jung and Campbell also helped me appreciate that myths are ancient stories that paradoxically depict *truths* beyond mere words or explanations. Just as parables convey truths beyond facts, myths transcend known material reality, extending into deeper meanings and immeasurable dimensions. With my worship of science and technology, I had previously dismissed the value of myths, mistakenly calling them falsehoods or reducing them to superstitions.

I gained a new respect for the ways symbols, myths, metaphors, archetypes, and parables access the larger mind, the unconscious. Symbols rarely make immediate sense to the rational mind; symbols require a different part of the mind in order to understand their meaning. While the conscious mind can often hide, run away from, shield, or deceive us about the meaning of our deeper selves, the unconscious mind simply presents images of truth that can guide us toward healing.

I often use the imagery from dreams to help people understand experiences they may be struggling with. John[10] was 37 years old when he was diagnosed with stomach cancer. He had a philosophical bent and was intrigued by symbols and dreams. He told me about a recurring nightmare he'd been having for the past several months. "This grotesque-looking travel agent keeps asking me what I want. I keep dodging her, but she always manages to find me. I wake up shaking in my skin."

"Next time you should ask her what she wants," I told him. I proposed that he try to meet her now, while he was awake and I was with him. "Close your eyes," I said quietly. "Bring her image to your mind." When he'd done that, I suggested that he tell her that next time she came, he was going to ask her what she wanted.

John sat quietly for a few moments before opening his eyes and nodding. "If you don't ask her in the dream," I said, "ask her as soon as you wake up. Stay in that twilight sleep of a relaxed frame of mind and ask her what she wants and then see what impressions come to mind."

A few weeks later, John came to tell me the travel agent had visited him in the night.

"What'd she tell you?" I asked, fascinated. I should have been prepared for his answer, but I wasn't.

"She said she wanted to help me get ready for my trip. She wanted me to be comfortable; she asked what I needed."

My heart sank as I realized what the trip would be, "How do you feel about what she told you?"

"Good. I'd never thought of her coming to *help* me. I only thought she was coming to take something away. Now I know I don't need to be afraid of her."

We then talked about what he needed to get ready for his "trip," focusing on end-of-life strategies that could prepare him.[11]

Our Hospice and Palliative Care unit also takes advantage of the power of symbols to help patients get in touch with the feelings they have about "getting ready for their trip." For example, in the hallway is a six-foot poster of an iceberg with views above and below the waterline. The meaning of the phrase, "the tip of the iceberg," is readily apparent as the massive ice structure beneath the ocean surface can be viewed objectively. Words that express various feelings are attached to the picture and can be moved with the invitation for the viewer to put words on the tip that reflect what they show on the surface. Likewise, words are selected to place on the iceberg's underneath surface to reflect what is kept hidden from view. The iceberg metaphor helps externalize what is sometimes difficult to articulate, helping us abide feelings we may not realize we have.

Clara, a veteran with cancer, was telling me that her family didn't want to hear anything except that things were getting better. She said her church community made her feel as if she had no faith when she voiced feelings of fear, anger, or pain. As she spoke, her voice was dull and lifeless. I showed her the iceberg poster. "Pick some words from the ice under the water and bring them up to the surface," I said, gesturing to the iceberg.

She surveyed the assortment, bringing a few words to the tip above the water. As she told me about the words, more emotions kept surfacing. By the time she finished, more feelings were above the waterline than there were spots to hold them. "I need to come back here every week so I can *see* what I'm feeling," she said with a laugh and lilt in her voice that reflected the vitality that had surfaced with her tears.

Clara reminded me that the vitality of expressing feelings can melt icebergs.

Patients often use metaphor to convey the status of their trip preparation. I asked a patient one day if he was ready for death should it come that day. He confidently replied, "I'm packed up, prayed up, and ready to go." I "high-fived" him and we relaxed in the satisfaction that nothing more need be done except open up to what was coming.

We use metaphors to help patients get packed up, prayed up, and ready to go, including paintings and murals. It started with a wall that had been temporarily erected in the hallway while some construction was going on nearby. We all hated it. We thought the cold, gray sheetrock interfered with the healing environment we tried to maintain. "Maybe some hospice graffiti would make it look better," one nurse suggested.

"Maybe we should put some furniture in front of it," said an aide.

"What about the painting we had made for our pins?" Sheila, a nurse on the unit, asked. That suggestion was it. We couldn't wait to get working on it. The pins she talked about were bought the year before when we had created a ceremony for new hospice staff. The ceremony included each person's receiving a tiny pin in the shape of three tiny footprints along with the words, "Know that your journey is sacred, and your footprints are holy." Then, each staff wrote their personal perspective of what their footprints pin symbolized for their role in helping people die healed. We then created a painting to depict the theme so patients would understand the meaning of the pins we wore.

It was a small painting, and we needed something to cover the whole ugly wall. We decided to reproduce it in an enlarged form. One evening, the hospice and palliative care physician brought paint and brushes. Through the night, Dr. Hull and the staff worked to reproduce the painting on the wall. One of our patients, Sydney, joined them. When difficulties with the re-creation of the rainbow were encountered, she had the solution. She wheeled back to her room and returned with some dental floss. "Now go get a tack and use my floss to draw the arc," she directed.

The next morning, Sydney asked a nurse to take her out to view the finished product. At first she just grinned at it, but then something moved her. Suddenly, years of uncried tears erupted into sobs. It was the first and only time Sydney surrendered to the pain of her experience. No one spoke. We sat with her as she cried, and when she looked back at us, her smile was peaceful.

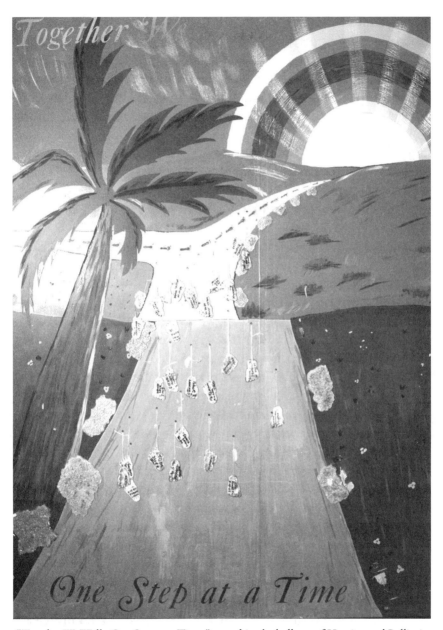

"Together We Walk, One Step at a Time," mural in the hallway of Hospice and Palliative Care unit.

The mural would come to have similar effects on others: family groups, employee bereavement groups, private patient sittings, and hospice staff on retreats. All found solace in the metaphorical image. "It's like a pathway to a new beginning," said one patient. "Everything levels off over the last hill and gets beautiful," a social worker commented. "The further along on the journey you go, the lighter it gets." One dying patient stared at it for a long while, then said, "I'm meeting my Maker, who is waiting to walk with me over the last hill, and than a new day is born."

Barbed Wire as a Metaphor for Our Lives

Prisoner of War (POW) camps for each war had their own cultures depending on the country they were in, the conditions they were subjected to, and the tortures used to extract information. I have heard horror stories from some of them. Perhaps most horrifying was the one told to me by a veteran who survived the Bataan Death march. As he and the other prisoners were walking past a field, a pregnant farm woman threw them some food she was picking. One of the guards walked over to her, pulled out his knife, and cut the baby out of her body as the helpless prisoners watched!

A few camps were humane; one allowed the prisoners to be more creative. It was Oflag 64 in Schubin, Poland. I learned about this camp from Russell Ford,[12] a veteran who had been diagnosed with depression. He seemed to be adjusting to his cancer easily enough, but he was desperately lonely. He was quite willing to talk about his life in the military, including the two and a half years he'd spent in the POW camp. When I asked him about some of his experiences I was surprised to see his face become intermittently animated. I was surprised because the details were unlike any I'd heard from other POWs. I encouraged him to consider writing down some of his memories.

"Oh, I already did that," he told me. Seven years after his release from the camp, he had found himself on a train going through Austria with a layover in Innsbruck. It triggered memories of the time he had traveled through Austria as a POW. "Only then it had been a *forced* stopover," he added with a dry laugh. He subsequently wrote a journal of those memories. At my request, he brought the journal to his next appointment. It was beautiful work, full of vivid images.

"I can still see the bombed-out houses in Berlin," one of his entries noted. "A kitchen might be entirely exposed with only one wall holding everything up. I could imagine how it would have been one minute before the bomb hit. The wife had probably just prepared lunch because the plates were still sitting on the table and the pot was still on the stove. The soup had boiled over; the dish towel still hung neatly over the sink. The hausfrau would never cook again."

"That's pretty chilling," I said repelled and fascinated at the same time.

"The only way America will ever become a peace-loving people is through a good taste of bombing and destruction," he had answered.

"I'm not sure I understand . . . "

"What do Americans really know about war?" he explained. "Do the Austrian people now want war? Of those that survived, do you think they now want war?"

"I hadn't thought about it before," I mused. "I would guess not."

After the war, Russell became a singer and producer of Broadway shows. His career, combined with his journal, gave me an idea.

"You've got to read this manuscript," I told my team members excitedly. "It's fascinating. It's a story that needs to be told. We could do Russell's life review like a play; we can make him think he's back on Broadway. I'll be the director and producer. You all can do the acting, and we'll do it as a dramatic reading so you can even read from the script. It'll be fun!"

My colleagues were persuaded easily enough. They knew the fulfillment of creative endeavors. I didn't tell Russ what we were plan-

ning; I only said it was something special for him. I also told him I
wanted him to prepare something to say about the lessons he'd
learned from his experiences as a POW so that he could pass those
lessons on to the rest of us.

I found a tape with military sound effects for artillery, aircraft,
and bombings so the audience could be acoustically sensitized to
POW life. One of Russell's visitors, who had been in the POW camp
with him, provided me with a live tape recording of the music they
had produced there. Talk about making the production authentic!

Production day arrived. We were ready, nervous, and eager.
Russell was brought to the auditorium in a wheelchair. He was given
a prominent view on the front row. Twenty volunteers and ten of
Russell's friends comprised the audience waiting to watch staff members enact his words.

I opened with a welcome that used the barbed wire of Russell's
POW experience as a metaphor for our own inner entrapments:
"Today is a special day because today you are going to hear a story.
It is the story of Russell Ford. Mr. Ford has a few months or so to
live. In hospice, we help people understand how their lives have
made a difference to the world. Russell's life has made a difference.
Telling his story connects his story to our own, for this is not just
Russell Ford's story. It's a story about *all* people. For in each of our
lives, in some way, we have felt trapped. All of us have been POWs
in some situations in which we lost our power. Each of us here has
faced circumstances that seemed to hold us prisoner without hope of
escape . . . circumstances that when we looked outward, all we could
experience was the barbed wire of our fear. When you look back
upon these circumstances and notice how you met the challenge . . .
how you overcame your feelings of powerlessness . . . how you
escaped in spite of the barbed wire of fear, you will notice that, just
as Russell Ford, you gained freedom from your fears . . . that somehow you faced the challenge and creatively met it. So the story you
will hear today is not just a remote piece of history that has little to
do with you. For when you look beyond the details, you will sense
the deeper meaning of the human spirit. You will realize that in some

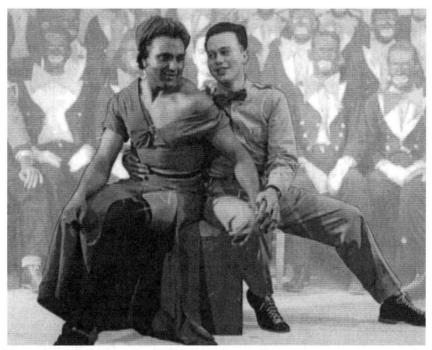

Russell Ford (left) in The Man Who Came to Dinner *performed at Oflag 64 POW camp.*

ways, you share in his invincibility. You share in his story."

The window shades were then dramatically lowered until the room blackened while *Fanfare for the Common Man* was played. Slides of Russell's prison camp were projected on a large screen as our "actors" read parts of Russell's journal. It was even more powerful read aloud than on the page; Russell's life had all the ingredients of pure drama. We began with his writings about his capture by German soldiers. "We hauled C rations and GI cans of water over the treacherous mountain passes," read hospice volunteer, Jim Donahue, dressed in his World War II uniform. "The Stuka dive bombers bombed our company with clocklike precision every day at 12:25 PM. We were frustrated with the orders that forbade us to fire back. On patrol one day, I unknowingly climbed into the middle of a German platoon. I used up all my ammunition, then hurled my gun over the mountain before surrendering. Meanwhile, a ricocheted bullet imbedded in my right leg, a testament to how bad a shot the Germans were."

The prisoners were then transported to the POW camp. They were marched to the train, but they defiantly refused to cower; they sang a hearty chorus of *I've Been Working on the Railroad* while anti-aircraft guns exploded like musical accompaniment. They paid no attention to the German guards' high-pitched, guttural order to "HALT! Dreizig men heringhr! Schnell!" Screaming men and women clutched their children hysterically.

They were then sealed into a boxcar where they remained for nearly a week. "Thirty of us crammed in the car with five loaves of dark bread and seven cans of horse meat," read John Hull, a physician on our hospice team. "The darkness kindly prevented us from seeing nervous sweating, the only sign of fear. Jokes covered up what we were 'sweating out.' What we were literally and figuratively 'sweating out' was life." Their only toilet was a bucket, which soon overflowed when the captives got diarrhea. The train stopped to pick up more captives, and the prisoners yelled out, asking the guards to open the door so the bucket could be emptied. They refused; but then one guard returned to open the door and ordered the soldiers to empty the bucket. When the prisoners then asked for water, the same guard brought it. "Were there good and bad enemies?" read Dr. Hull. "Would this man, who had taken pity on us, possibly at considerable personal risk, be condemned for his act of mercy? I searched for answers, only to find more questions."

At the camp, now living with 1600 other prisoners, Russell and his comrades suffered relentless hunger pangs. Weak soup, a few potatoes, and turnips that invariably had stuck to the bottom of the cooking pot were their only food. "I can never forget the fierce taste of burned horse turnips," Russell had written. Dysentery was common, but any attempt to go to the latrine at night was interpreted as an escape and was met with a volley of bullets.

The prisoners were determined to survive, both physically and psychically. They played baseball and football, and even held a track and field competition. "But the Germans objected to our cross-country proposal," Russell had written. "Imagine 1600 inmates on the run over the countryside!" Prisoners with expertise in a subject became camp "professors" teaching classes in accounting, language arts, animal husbandry, botany, and art. Russell's own expertise was theatre and he decided to put on a zany comedy that had been popular in America, *The Man Who Came to Dinner*.[13] They fashioned a stage from foraged lumber with powdered milk tins for reflectors. Burlap bags were torn up to make bust pads for the female roles. "We got makeup by bribing the German officers," read Chaplain Dan in a high-pitched voice as he impersonated Russell as he had appeared on stage attired in a dress, wig, makeup, high heels, and carrying a purse.

The play was so popular that they did other plays every month and started a weekly glee club and variety show. The guards loved the shows and got instruments for the prisoners. "However the guards were puzzled by the 'Let's go Ike' signs held up by the cast at the end of shows."

For Russell, not only surviving but thriving became a source of pride. "Camp life had different meanings for different prisoners," he had written. "For some, it had been a torture. For others, it had been a vacuum. For myself, in some ways, it had been rewarding. Everything we had done had been accomplished in spite of lack of food. Every prisoner had a chance to find himself through activities, examine himself as a person, and enter communal life. Most prisoners did this successfully for themselves, for their peace of mind, and for their future. For me, camp life had been a lesson in 'community'."

In the final scene, Russell's reflections from his diary were read. "We had been a generation of young men who had been born just after World War I, grown up in the wild 1920s, suffered the poverty of the nation's greatest depression, and came to manhood just in time to be drafted into war. Our reward for winning the war had been some medals and artificial limbs. For others, it was a white cross on a field. For the remainder, it was a confusing and perplexing world. Didn't Alexander the Great cross the same Atlas Mountains in Africa with his legions that I crossed with mine? Yet, Alexander the Great's civilization decayed and fell. Would our atom bomb that replaced his spears bring a new and lasting peace? It's a question I often ponder . . . "

The lights slowly came up. Russell remained spellbound, even in his applause. A staff member escorted him to the microphone. With strength and animation I'd not seen from him before, he thanked us for the production and then read the message he had prepared:

> I've long wanted to tell people what I felt about the progress we may have made since the war. If we've made any progress in the last 50 years, it doesn't show as brightly as I had hoped. I hope in the next 50 years, we'll gather our souls together and ourselves together and make an America that is totally one nation, indivisible. Indivisible means you cannot, therefore will not, have different races. You have one race . . . one love of mankind.
>
> And love . . . love is the only thing that will keep our life and souls and families together. We need love all over the world, not just here in the United States. Love that goes on day by day. Love that is permanent cannot be rejected. Love cannot be forgotten. Love is the glue of generations, the cement of civilizations. It is the span between life and death. Love must be the salvation of nations, the only cornerstone on which the future can endure. For love alone will outlast any enemy or any war. Love is what we will build our lives on. Love is what God is, and in the end, it's all we have and all I leave to you, my good friends, is love . . .

Accessing the Lessons of the Crescent Moon Bear

- Veterans who have recovered from the trials in their lives by gradually awakening deeper dimensions within themselves can inspire us to want to grow and change.
- It takes courage to let go of our fears and instead show up for things in our lives we'd prefer to fight, flight, or freeze. It requires honesty to let go of illusions, denials, and pretenses so that we can open up to our authentic self, including those aspects of ourselves we'd prefer to hide. Paradoxically, humility empowers us; we gain real power when we let go of pride and will power and open up to acknowledge our needs and ask for help.
- People who have met their Crescent Moon Bear know how to abide and reckon with walled-off pieces of self and integrate suffering instead of run from it. They have a peace beyond worldly understanding.
- Retrieving fragments of scattered, hidden selves is the task after trauma.
- When people are dying, their conscious mind recedes and their unconscious mind expands; the language of the unconscious is symbols and images.
- Symbols speak what words cannot, awakening us to dimensions words can't reach. Symbols touch the larger self.
- Myths are ancient stories that paradoxically depict truths beyond mere words or explanations.
- While the conscious mind can often hide, run away from, shield, or deceive us about the meaning of our deeper selves, the unconscious mind simply presents images of truth that can guide us toward healing.
- Love is what God is and in the end, it's all we have and all I leave to you.

Chapter Eight

The Life I Never Anticipated

May each of us have the Grit, the Grace, the Humility, the Love
to heal our war-ravaged soldiers and our broken nation.
May we be the link that connects the circle so they
feel connected to Humanity once again.
May we not miss the opportunity to help these
veterans recover their souls from
Iraq   Desert Storm   Vietnam   Korea   Nazi Germany
and various other parts of the world where they served
so they can have peace . . . at last.
May we help them know that the circle goes on, joining
them to you and to me.
Our people, our nation, our God
would be ever so grateful.[1]

When I started writing this book, I said that I had never anticipated the life I ended up having. Yet as I'm completing the book, it occurs to me that in some ways this life really hasn't been so unanticipated after all. In Chapter 2, I wrote about a night 15 years ago when Vietnam veteran, Tommy Bills, sat at my table eating dinner with my husband and me. At that table, I had said, "Our *whole* nation needs healing. Our nation's *soul* needs healing." It was as much a prayer as it was an explanation. A shiver had gone up my spine as I had spoken the words. Maybe my career has simply been an answer to that prayer. As I look at the Vietnam service bars those two veterans gave me 15 years ago, I sometimes wonder if I wasn't being drafted into this unanticipated life, and on some level, I accepted the mission without knowing it. I'm grateful I did; I've been the recipient of veteran wisdom. I heard about a tradition an African tribe uses to express gratitude to someone who has done something a tribesman appreciates. The tribesman goes to that person's doorstep and sits with his forehead on the ground. Sometimes, I have an urge to place my forehead on the floor of our Hospice and Palliative Care unit to pay homage to all the gifts my veterans have given me.

I have tried to share the lessons my veterans have taught me. Most people are very compassionate and eager to learn, but they often have some reluctance.

"I want to try some of these things you're talking about, but I fear opening up a can of worms that I can't put back." It's a statement I've heard more than once. People fear asking about war, death, trauma, "negative" feelings; they don't know what the question will trigger.

"Open yourself to the person. *Want* to hear them," I say. "Be willing to ask the difficult questions that no one else asks. Ask about the worms. If they don't want to bring out any worms, respect that and don't push them; but when the worms do come out, don't be afraid of them. Ask the person to describe the worms. Ask them to feel the worms. Feel the worms with them. Tell them you're sorry they've had such a wormy experience. Ask them what they want to do with the worms today and how you can be helpful. Tell them you appreciate their honesty in acknowledging their worms, their courage in opening the can, and their humility in asking for help to bring the worms out in the open so they can be used to aerate the soil." I always remind people that the most effective and authentic way to help others with their worms is for them to practice abiding and reckoning with their own worms. "We can't help others touch their worms if we don't know how to abide and reckon with our own." The paradox is that once we do that, we can then go fishing with our worms to help others.[2]

I think our concerns also stem from an under-appreciation of how strong veteran worm-bearers are. Respecting how fast and how many worms people want to bring out of the can allows them to control the can-opening process. They bring out what they are ready to reckon with at that time. What they are not ready for will remain stuffed or hidden; suppression and denial are important protective mechanisms that serve as natural gatekeepers for what we are not yet willing, able, or ready to reckon with. The goal is not necessarily to put the worms back where they were nor is it our job; it's the veteran's job. There's often a bit of struggle involved in figuring out what to do with worms once they've come out. That's okay. Struggle is what often moves people to deeper levels within themselves to discover lessons not previously experienced. Encouraging them in deep breathing can help them abide and reckon with their experience so they can stay in the discomfort of the moment.

I think another fear of opening cans of worms is that medical textbooks and training often devote much time and attention to controlling, containing, and coping with out-of-can worms. These processes are important and necessary, but attention also needs to be paid to abiding and reckoning with the worms. My emphasis on the latter doesn't mean I don't value the former; I hope peoples' fears about the latter don't keep them from becoming can openers. I believe we do harm forcing cans of worms open when people don't want or aren't ready to have them opened. I also believe we do harm by not offering options to open the can; that's called abandonment. Patients may not realize they have cans that need opening. Even if they know the worms are there, they may not realize the value of opening the can.

The lessons I've learned about opening cans of worms are both similar to, and different from, lessons nonveteran patients provide to their caregivers. It was an innocent conversation among my non-VA hospice colleagues that made me realize how veterans sometimes have a different experience of death than nonveterans. My non-VA colleagues were eager to hear how stoicism, PTSD, and fight/flight/freeze behaviors sometimes interfere with peaceful dying. "We don't know these things. You need to teach us," two community hospice executives told me. Since 1800 veterans are dying every day (25% of all Americans who are dying in 2009) and 96% of these veterans die outside the VA system, much of the information seemed highly relevant.[3,4] The funny thing was, I didn't realize I knew these

things either. Having worked for the VA my entire career, veterans
were all I knew. When I was asked to do a presentation about hospice care for veterans at the Florida Hospice-Veterans Partnership
meeting,[5] I was forced to articulate concepts and patterns of behavior I'd observed over the years.

Since then, I've traveled the country doing presentations for
staff at VAs, community hospices, and professional conferences.
Entitled "Wounded Warriors: Their Last Battle," the presentations
are about the concepts I have articulated in this book. The presentation has even been televised and reproduced on DVD. I've been
stunned by the response. I think there are two reasons why the presentations have been met with such enthusiasm. I'm told my observations about veterans are original. No one had previously thought
about the effects of war on peoples' experience of death, not even
PTSD healthcare providers or hospice workers. I also think my message has been embraced because what I speak about is not wholly
original. I speak about how to respond to stoicism, guilt-laden war-
induced memories, alcohol-numbing at end of life, and the wisdom
our warriors have to share when we open up to their lessons.
Audiences nod their heads in agreement because they recognize their
own veteran patients or family members they've cared for; my message resonates with what they already know. I've come to realize that
I'm not introducing any new dots; I'm just connecting dots.

I've been humbled by the veterans who have come up after presentations to express their gratitude for my acknowledgement of
their military service. Vietnam veterans and their families often
thank me for acknowledging what has often previously gone unacknowledged. One man tearfully said, "My Dad would want me to
thank you for what you said today. He was killed in Vietnam." I
could only share his tears as I hugged that soldier's son and imagined
a little boy who had lost his hero father to our nation and the suffering that loss had caused him.

Many veterans appreciate shedding light on their postmilitary
struggles. Some have come to tell me they recognized symptoms of
PTSD in themselves. Hundreds of combat veterans have told me the

equivalent of "I want you to know you have opened a door that is starting my healing." Families of Iraq war veterans poignantly ask, "How can I prevent this with my young soldier?" I always encourage them to seek help at Vet Centers. I know that these soldiers also have a hero within that will lead them out of darkness into the light of themselves. I also know that it's not an easy journey and that reaching out for help increases the likelihood of success.

Wives and ex-wives have come forward to say they were enlightened about PTSD. "My husband is a combat veteran. I've seen these behaviors. It all makes sense now. I've got to tell my adult children about this so they understand some of their father's actions when they were young." One woman in Nebraska, Theresa Wood, told me that all five of her mother's brothers had gone to Vietnam. She became so impassioned about what she learned that she launched a coalition in her community to raise awareness of veterans' issues at end of life.

A few citizens have come forward to confess their callousness in ignoring the plight of returning combat veterans. "I didn't spit on them when they returned from Vietnam, but I'm ashamed to say I turned my back on them. Now, I'm going to go to Washington, D.C. to the Vietnam Wall and touch their names and ask their forgiveness," one woman told me.

I've received hundreds of e-mails from people telling me how veterans have benefited from interventions I had suggested. One nurse in South Carolina, Sharon Hutch, tells of a patient who was a Vietnam veteran. He had a lot of pain and refused all help. He couldn't even sleep. She writes:

> After hearing you speak, I realized the importance of acknowledging his military service. The next time I visited him, I thanked him for all he had done for our country and acknowledged what it had cost him. He cried and cried, saying no one had ever thanked him. He had three times previously refused to see our chaplain, but now asked

for him. When the chaplain came, the patient spoke to him about dreams in which animal-like people were chasing him and making him do things he didn't want to do. He said he had been refusing the medications because he was afraid to sleep and have the dreams come back. Since talking with the chaplain about the dreams, the dreams have stopped. He's now resting and lies peacefully in his son's home. I don't think he'll live beyond today, but I know his spirit is free and his eyes no longer have that wild, haunted look.

Asian healthcare providers sometimes attend my presentations. They thank me for helping them understand how their heritage can act as a trigger with Vietnam, Korean, and Pacific theater World War II veterans. They realize they need not take it personally; neither does it necessarily mean the veteran is racist. One e-mail from a physician notes, "I was able to help one of my hospice patients who was having flashbacks of Vietnam triggered by my Asian heritage. Because of what I learned from your talk, I was able to bring him home from that flashback."

Many VA staff talk about how the presentation awakens them to the needs of veterans. One physician at a VA clinic tearfully told me, "I've been here for two years and there are many days when I ask myself, 'Why am I doing this? I don't understand these guys.' You've helped me understand who these veterans are and what they need."

A physician from a state veterans' nursing home excitedly told me how he had admitted a difficult patient. "He was agitated, confused, and demanding. Other nursing homes had turned this patient down. But after watching your DVD, our staff recognized that it was PTSD. They feel so satisfied to know they've been able to respond to his wartime wounds."

A community inpatient hospice told me they redecorated one unit with military décor, placing only veterans on that unit. This allows the "brotherhood"/"sisterhood" to develop, common stories to be told, and appreciation for each other's service to be expressed. Many hospices, including our own, recognize the value of having double rooms for veterans on inpatient units. There is therapeutic power between dying veterans; they en-courage and comfort one another in ways that no one else can. Some hospices have started programs whereby those of their volunteers who are veterans are assigned to veteran patients so camaraderie is fostered. Almost all community hospices are now asking patients on admission if they are veterans. Many hospices now provide certificates recognizing military service. Some require all employees to watch the DVD of *Wounded Warriors* to improve their care for veterans. The follow-up training DVD is then utilized to help them develop skills in caring for veterans who are nearing the end of their lives.[6] Hopefully they will also require them to read this book.

I've also had some negative encounters. One related to anger at the VA for not diagnosing cancer at an earlier stage. Another was from an atheist who protested I had used the word "God." One questioned my credibility, "Only veterans should be talking about veteran issues." I've had a few PTSD professionals who questioned some of my experiences and responses to patients with PTSD. When I remind them that the experience of PTSD can change dramatically as people are dying, however, they immediately grasp the significance; PTSD professionals simply have not had the opportunity to bear witness to patients as they die or do not have the experience of new-onset PTSD that presents at the end of life.

I'm sure there will be more criticism, some deserved and some not. I hope I will be able to stay open to both and be able to discern the difference. With one criticism, I had to discern that difference quickly because it happened publicly. I conclude my *Wounded Warrior: Their Last Battle* presentation by having the veterans in the audience stand. Staff then pin each of them with an American flag pin that says "Honored Veteran." One time, I failed to bring enough pins and so some veterans were left out. After all sat down, a veteran raised his hand. He was red in the face and his speech was both halting and urgent. "I'm so pissed off right now, I don't even know if I can talk," he blurted out. I could only wait anxiously while he collected his thoughts. "I'm a Vietnam veteran. I didn't get a pin. Once again, I'm pushed to the side. This is exactly what happened when I came back home 40 years ago." His next words were heartbreaking. Tearfully he asked, "When is it going to end?"

Initially, I was speechless; my heart sank as I felt this man's betrayal. The very thing I had hoped to accomplish (bring healing, hope, and homecoming to our vets) had produced just the opposite effect. "I am so sorry, sir," I said sincerely. "I don't know what I can say to make it up to you. The last thing I would want to do is push you aside."

"It's a little too late for that," he said sarcastically.

A veteran from the other side of the room came over to him. She took her pin off that she had just received and pinned it on him. "I want you to have this. You deserve it more than I do." The room erupted into applause, but it didn't stop there. Shirl, one of my colleagues, came over to him.

"I was one of those people who pushed you aside 40 years ago," she said. "I was a Vietnam War protester in the 60s." He looked at her guardedly before she explained. "My brother was in Vietnam, and I was doing what I could to bring him home."

"You don't know how much that hurt us," he said plaintively.

"You're right. I didn't," Shirl responded tenderly. "But I do now and I'm sorry I hurt you." Tears and hugs sealed their reconciliation while the room burst into applause yet again.

"This is how we heal our nation," I told the audience. "One soldier at a time . . . one gratitude at a time . . . one apology at a time . . ."

Final Lessons Learned?

- Open yourself to the person. *Want* to hear them.
- Be willing to ask the difficult questions that no one else asks. Ask about the worms.
- If they don't want to talk about the worms, respect that. Don't force them or make them feel guilty if they choose to keep the worms in the can. There are times when the can is the best place for them.
- When the worms come out, don't be afraid of them. Ask the person to describe the worms.
- Ask them to feel the worms. Feel the worms with them.
- Tell them you're sorry they've had such a wormy experience.
- Ask them what they want to do with the worms today and how you can be helpful.
- Tell them you appreciate their honesty in acknowledging their worms, their courage in opening the can, and their humility in asking for help to bring the worms out in the open so they can be used to aerate the soil.
- Practice abiding and reckoning with your own worms. Then use them to go fishing.
- We heal our nation one soldier at a time . . . one gratitude at a time . . . one apology at a time.

Epilogue

It was Thomas Edes MD, Chief of Home and Community Based Care for the Department of Veterans Affairs in Washington, D.C. who first recognized the importance of the message I was delivering about my observations related to veterans' deaths. "No one has talked or written about these things before. We've got to get this message out," he told me. Shortly thereafter, he arranged a broadcast on the subject to VAs throughout the country, along with a DVD reproduction. Since then, my life has not been the same.

Sometimes it's hard for me to believe I've become a public speaker. Like most people, I've had to overcome a dreadful fear of it. Telling myself, "It's not about you, Deborah; it's about the veterans. Just share your passion" has pushed me beyond my ego so I can let go of fear of judgment and criticism and open up to grace and mercy.

I've had to overcome my ineptitude with computers and media products.[1] The transparencies I used on an overhead projector got replaced last year with Power Point computerized programs, much to my protests. I also learned that it's best to remove a portable microphone prior to going into the bathroom if you don't want your private business a public affair!

I've had many expected and unexpected pleasures. In my presentation, I speak about metaphor, citing the book *Final Gifts*[2] by two hospice nurses, Pat Kelley and Maggie Callanan. After a presentation in Boston, a woman came forward to introduce herself.

"My name is Pat Kelley," she said.

I didn't comprehend the significance. (I mean Pat Kelley is a common name. What are the odds that the one I spoke about during the presentation is the one in front of me?).

"The *Final Gifts* Pat Kelley," she clarified.

"Oh my Gosh!" I exclaimed, hugging her.

I was also fortuned to meet Florence Wald, the director of the first hospice in America when I went to Connecticut. How validating it was for me to receive her endorsement! We both cried.

I was also pleased to renew my friendship with Tommy Bills, the

first "wounded warrior" who I wrote about in Chapter 2. I was presenting in south Florida and invited him to attend. I hadn't seen him
since our original encounter 15 years earlier. I had no trouble recognizing him even though his ponytail was gone. At the end of the
presentation, with his painting displayed on the projected screen, I
called him up on stage. It was a moment to behold.

Mostly I've met people who have not been famous. They've been
ordinary people providing extraordinary service. Meeting them has
been life-giving. It has awakened my appreciation for the men and
women who have dedicated their lives to "serving those who first
served us." For many, working in the VA is a life devoted to bringing
our soldier's back "in one piece," even if it occurs one piece at a time.
These staff strive to understand the impact military life causes, working tirelessly and unceasingly to restore wholeness. They often work
behind the scenes. Many are veterans and provide service from a personal understanding. Many have never been a veteran; they serve
from a willingness to listen and be changed by what they hear. I've
also been fortunate to meet hospice colleagues who do not work for
the VA. They have rallied around this work, recognizing and supporting the homecoming each veteran deserves. These are the people
I've had the privilege of meeting in my travels around the country.

Having little wanderlust, I never anticipated the travel I've
embarked upon. I've always enjoyed my home, work, and family.
Speaking trips became necessary interruptions threatening my con-
tentment. As I realized my resentment, I knew I needed to change
my relationship to traveling. I started asking colleagues to accompany me, turning a travel obligation into an adventure, an opportunity to explore this country and its people.

When I drive, I stay off interstate roads. It's hard to experience
the country on an interstate road; each state looks the same, their
inhabitants remain unmet and untouched. Everything is predictable;
speed and destination the goals. There are few cars on the back roads;
they're all on the interstate roads which mean time is not excessively
lost. On the back roads, I've discovered parks, golf courses, and veteran memorials. I found "Useless Cemetery" in Missouri and "Coon

Dog Cemetery" in Alabama and a Chinese restaurant that specializes in American barbeque in Arizona. They each became uproarious adventures.

On one of my adventures, my travel companion brought a computerized mapping system. With a punch of a button, a voice tells you every turn to arrive at your destination. "No. No. No," I had protested. "That interferes with the surprise and adventure. Searching it out and getting lost are part of the fun."

Surprisingly, I've seldom gotten lost. Maps and signs still work remarkably well in and between most cities, except Boston. Boston has its own rules and its own way of doing signs (or not doing them). They also have confusing intersections called "jug handles" where you turn right in order to go left and vice versa.

I inadvertently became part of the annual "Balloon Parade" in Iowa. I just waved and acted like I belonged. No one knew the difference. Everyone welcomes you in Iowa, even if you don't belong. This year the parade focused on supporting the troops in Iraq. I was raised in the cornfields of Indiana. I'm not naïve to farm culture, but did you know they name their tractors in Iowa? To a person who named her cat "Cat," this was indeed a marvel.

Illinois has cities like Oblong and Green Up. If you don't know where they are, go to Bone Gap and take a left. Be careful though. There's a lot of construction there. Signs warn you that speeding fines are doubled unless you hit a worker. The sign says that hitting a construction worker will cost you $10,000.

The Midwest is filled with licks . . . Mayslick, Gum Lick, French Lick and Licking River; and if you haven't eaten fresh deep-fried cheese curds from Wisconsin cheese factories, you don't know what you're missing!

I've jogged and done yoga on beaches and deserts with suns setting and moons rising. I visited New Orleans the week before Hurricane Katrina visited. I stayed in the hotel next to the Superdome, the one with all the windows gone that was in many of the broadcasts. It made the scenes more real and surreal for me. New Orleans made me realize that meeting and loving people means you meet and grieve their trauma as well. Most of my new friends at the New Orleans VA did not fare well.

Traveling has also forced me to confront my prejudices. Born in the Midwest and moving to Florida when I became an adult, travel was limited to visiting family. Other than my trip to India, I had only known the down-to-earth attitudes of Midwesterners and the charm of the South. I'd harbored a prejudice against Northerners. Secretly, I'd held onto beliefs that big city Northerners were rude, merciless, and obnoxious. They crowded my already crowded roads in Florida in the wintertime.

I've had to change those beliefs.

"The South has nothing over you guys," I sincerely told my gracious and generous Northern hosts. They can't appreciate the hidden surprise with which I say it, or maybe they can. It's hard to hide prejudices.

Traveling has meant other unanticipated changes, like letting go of some of my patient responsibilities. My colleagues also complain about my absence. "You're never here anymore," they sometimes grumble to my already guilt-ridden ears. I began to question my new role. Though I had received much collegial acclaim which was satisfying, I saw fewer patients, which was proportionately less satisfying. I questioned my new role, praying for guidance. The next day a patient who had frequented my office whenever he was admitted to the hospital came to see me. He said he'd come several times over the past few months but I'd not been there.

"The staff here say you're on the road all the time now."

"Yeah. It's true," I said bracing myself for another onslaught of "you've abandoned us" comments.

Instead, he said, "I'm so glad to hear that. Others need to learn how to help patients the way you do."

After he left, I looked upward, saying, "Okay. I accept."

Yet Another Unanticipation

Public speaking has not been the only change I've had to reckon with. I was doing a presentation in New York City. Afterwards a distinguished gentleman approached me, introducing himself as Dan Tobin. I recognized his name from his book, *Peaceful Dying*.[3] I was shocked by Dr. Tobin's question for me.

"Would you consider writing a book?"

I politely declined.

"I think you're onto something with the things you're saying. I'd like to help you get this message out."

I remained hesitant. "I like to write, but I'm not a writer." He encouraged me not to let that stop me. Over the ensuing months, with his encouragement, I was able to change my mind.

I've discovered the lonely life of a writer, the long hours in front of a computer and the tense neck and shoulder muscles that accompany it. I write in my home, a home bought from the widow of a Korean War veteran who committed suicide. Somehow it seems fitting. Maybe his suffering is somehow redeemed from these walls as I give voice to his despair.

I hope I've not portrayed myself as an island. I'm part of a team who struggles together with our humanity as we openly struggle with our patients' suffering. We're a team who isn't afraid to struggle with difficult patients. In fact, most of the stories in this book are memorable because of the struggle. There is synergy in a team. There is communion. Though I will be identified as the author, this book is the product of a group experience. I'm also fortunate to have small communities of friends who abide and help me reckon with personal struggles.

I've gone to great strides to preserve the accuracy and integrity of each story. I'm thankful I had written several stories years ago as they occurred so I could use them for teaching purposes. With others, I was able to view the medical record, thankful my documentation was complete and filled with patient quotes. For some stories, I've made calls to patient's family members to confirm details and memories. That has brought some welcome reunions.

I hope I've been able to resist the urge to embellish stories or manipulate them to meet personal needs. Nevertheless, I recognize my memory has the filter of my mind which can only alter facts and perspectives. Even though I aspire to know "the truth" because I know it will "set me free," I'm not foolish enough to think I don't suffer my humanity.

I've learned about reconciling the discipline of writing when I don't feel like it with waiting for the spirit-filled "zone" that sometimes descends seemingly out of nowhere. I've learned how grueling and creative it can be to craft a single paragraph and the hours it takes to do it. I've suffered the turned-down invitations of family and friends as my nonwriting life has been put on hold.

"I'll be glad when I get my life back," I keep saying while my gardens become a wasteland; my house grows thick with dust. At the same time, I'll miss the daily companionship with this material. I'll miss the relationship with you who are going to read this. Though you haven't met me until you picked up this book, believe me I've met you over the four years it has taken to write it. I sit with your anticipated needs always on my heart. "Will they want to know this? Do I need to take this out because it'll bore them? Will they care about this or is it mainly something I care about? Am I meeting their needs or projecting my own?"

On and on I go hoping I've sensed your needs. Though our relationship may never physically materialize, it is a relationship that is no less real. It is also a relationship that I now need to let go of so I can open up to a different future. May we each go forward with a renewed determination to show up openheartedly to our lives so we can become the hero we want to be and others need us to become.[4]

Appendix A

Tommy Bill's Diary

This appendix provides the reader with Tommy's complete diary. He wrote it 20 years after the war was over as part of his recovery process. Just as Tommy's painting had awakened my soul, this diary awakened my mind. It filled in the blanks of ignorance I had maintained.

After Tommy's diary, I have included my own journal entry. I mailed it to Tommy because I wanted him to know how his story had changed me. Looking back, it's easy to see how the formation of this book has its roots in that initial crude attempt to understand "wounded warriors" and learn how to "walk in the woods" with them.

I would also refer the reader to an excellent book entitled, *Visions of War, Dreams of Peace,* for further reading about recovery from war.[1] It is a collection of poems written by women who served in Vietnam. Its eye-opening contents make the struggle to reckon with the aftermath of war very real. I've included excerpts from a few short poems at the end of the appendix.

The following is Tommy Bill's diary:

It was sometime in 1965 . . . the latter part of the year. There was this tea plantation by Pleiku. The convoy drove through the place where those Green Berets held out for so long. My God . . . there were skeletons everywhere! Even the jeeps had skulls on their hoods . . . until the Colonel ordered their removal. I could feel their ghosts.

I was digging a foxhole out on the perimeter. Then I was told the fire team leader was to take my place because I was needed to stay near the jeep. If we were hit, I was to spirit the Colonel away. I left my foxhole and went over to the aide tent to see what was going on. A doctor told me to hold a compression bandage on the sucking chest wound of a young soldier who had a neat, round hole in the middle of his chest.

The doctor told me I was to keep my charge occupied "over there" because there were others who might still "make it" that he needed to work on. I kept assuring the sucking chest wound attached to the desperate soldier that we had the best medics anywhere . . . that these were the doctors that would help the Colonel if he were shot.

For just a moment, I let myself look beyond the gaping and the sucking. He had an all-American face and body. He had to have been my age—maybe even younger. No hair on his chest. Maybe he didn't even shave every day yet. A solid build . . . probably played some football in high school.

The air gurgled in and out more loudly. With renewed determination, I increased my pressure on the bandage. If I pressed hard enough, surely I could make it stop. The gurgling became more muffled but no amount of pressure could muffle his pleas. He called out for his mother; he called out for God. Grabbing my arms, he pleaded, "Please don't let me die" . . . not just once . . . not just twice . . . but, over and over again. Each desperate plea increased my own desperation.

I can't remember if I actually called to the doctors for help. I remember more wounded brought in . . . one after the other. I remember the doctor telling me to "just keep him quiet so he doesn't upset the others too much." I don't know (and don't know if I want to know) whether he died then or just passed out, but they carried him away. Part of me wanted frantically to be carried away too.

There was still shooting around us. I remember crawling out of the building and seeing the Sergeant-Major sitting on my jeep—just sitting out in the open with all this firing going on. I made my way to him to see if he knew the name of the guy I had been caring for.

"Doesn't matter," he told me. "There'll be lots more dying before this is over."

The next day, we loaded several body bags into choppers. My fire team leader who had taken my place in the foxhole was one of them. I was told he was the first one to die with the initial incoming round—it had hit right on my foxhole. Another bag held a body whose chest wound was no longer sucking . . . at least for him . . . because it was still sucking and gurgling in *my* mind.

Over the years, my memories have been of the contents of those two bags: the fire team leader who had taken my place in the foxhole who was the first to die as well as the guy who so desperately pleaded with me to not let him die . . . who also died. Maybe these two memories were all my mind could handle. Maybe there are other memories that had to be shut out.

I do still have vague memories of the convoys . . . the dust of the roads . . . the kids lining the streets with their hands out for C-rations we would throw to them . . . the four-year-old kids with cigarettes in their mouths—trying to see if we would pay to screw their sisters, their middle fingers pointing skyward, the few words they could speak in English: "Fuck you GI" . . . the kid they wired and sent up to the convoy—the explosion took out four of us, but the kid . . . I can't forget that kid blowing up!

In my letters home, I told my family it was like camping out in south Florida when I was a kid. Can you believe it? I actually told them there was enjoyment in doing what I did! God, I was good. I led everyone to believe I was so well-adjusted.

I still have trouble remembering the time we got hit in the field. That was the one and only time I got stoned. It was the place where we captured two Viet Cong and hung them up in camp. They were dead and some guys were having target practice with their knives. They told me to get up closer to have a look, but I found some reason to go to the other end of the compound. It would be many years before I could "get up closer to have a look" at any of my experiences . . . or any of my feelings . . . or just about any other part of "me." I could always find a reason to "go to the other end." I could always find a reason to run and hide from myself. I was so afraid—not that I would have admitted it. You see, on a military base, what everyone says is "It don't mean nothin"—as we struggled to shut out those "nothins" we were feeling.

One of those "nothins" I'm supposed to not feel was the unforgivable actions of one of my officers. He ordered that we take this hill that had no strategic significance; he knew the Vietcong body count would be higher than our own; this would show his combat prowess so he could gain a promotion. And as if that wasn't bad enough, we'd then be ordered to abandon the hill, so he could do it again—and even a third time! If any of us would have reported him, we would have been shot. I shudder every time I think of the lives sacrificed—all for his glory. But, I lock this up too. Some people call it "the thousand yard stare;" I call it "puttin' on the face," and I became very good at it. I built a wall like Ft. Knox: it was easy to make deposits but seemingly impossible to retrieve anything from behind it.

It wasn't just on a military base I was taught to not feel what I was feeling. In my family, we were to hide our feelings under a stoic mask of "I can handle anything because I'm a man." I would start to feel what was happening and shove those feelings down . . . doing what I saw everyone else doing. I wasn't going to be called a "sissy" or a "chicken." My father was a World War II veteran. I was raised on John Wayne movies. Pilgrims, settlers, adventurers, and soldiers were examples of what a man was to be.

When I was nine years old, I was told I would now be allowed the privilege of standing in the duck blind with a shotgun alongside my Dad. I anticipated this rite of passage with fear and loathing, yet acted as if I were delighted. When I knocked down my first bird, I was praised . . . and I died a little inside. As I was shooting, I was concentrating on hitting a moving object—like in skeet practice. So, I shot the "skeet" and plucked its feathers and ate it when we cooked it. That was when my concentration shifted into not feeling anything about what was really happening.

As I grew up, I felt confused and conflicted about animals (because some you loved and cared for and others you shot) and about how to "act" when I was hurt, sorry, glad, or sad. As a teenager, I discovered alcohol was a good anesthetic. Numbing feelings was a good prerequisite for Vietnam. It was in Vietnam that the myths blew up—though that didn't keep me from "shoulding" all over myself (about how I "should" have acted and reacted).

In Vietnam, all of the hunting and killing I'd learned over the years took on a whole new perspective. The "animals" I was supposed to kill were two-legged "animals" and I'm taught new names for them—"gook," "slant," "cong," "slope," anything that sounds less human. And now, there's an animal who can kill me!

But when I let myself really look, I see a simple Vietnamese people who just wanted to be left alone so they could tend their rice fields. I was thrown into contact with these "people" (can they be "people" during the day and "gooks" and "animals" at night?). They, too, were trying hard not to show their feelings (and failing). Shooting small birds and my military training just haven't prepared me for this.

A part of me thanks God I had the early training to block out the bad stuff . . . and a part of me is terribly sad I missed all of those opportunities to be "real." But I'm not sure I'd even be here today if I had a slip of "being real" while on the battlefield.

When did my "loss of innocence" begin? As an infant watching the "big boys" and my male role models? At nine years old in the duck blind? At 19 in the boat to Vietnam? At 20 holding a dying youth my own age? At 25 with my first wife or 35 with my second or 45 with my third?

Twenty-five years after the war, I'm still piecing together all of the damage done. I came back to a country who didn't know what to do with me. The Veteran's of Foreign Wars wouldn't even let me join: "Vietnam wasn't a real war," I was told. That cut me like a knife. But now I'm able and willing to look at what society, family, peers, and the military has done to a shy, sensitive kid who just wanted to like everyone and have everyone like him.

Between marriages, drug and alcohol addictions, homelessness, and bouts with liver disease that brought me to death's door a few times, I began to dabble in art and sculpture. On the surface, the images didn't seem to have anything to do with war. It wasn't until several years later that a psychologist viewing my artwork, saw what it was hiding. With his help, as well as the support from a Vietnam Veteran group, I began to let these paintings and sculptures emerge naturally and uninhibited. And what gradually revealed itself was Vietnam. This time, I let myself feel my trauma . . . the fear . . . the pain . . . the anger . . . the helplessness . . . the loneliness . . . the guilt . . . the uncertainty. And I began to heal.

Now, I can really feel what happened to me as a child, as a soldier, and what is happening to me as a man. With this freedom, comes the ability to laugh and cry . . . to be playful and happy and be me naturally. Now, I've had the walk in the woods with the wounded warriors.

My Own Journal Entry that I Mailed to Tommy

"Dysfunctional vets bear no scars, you know" my shallow selves jeer . . .
  My deeper self counters that
    these soldiers' wounds are much deeper.
Shallow selves persist: "No one can see their wounds.
  The doctor can't measure the wound.
  Where is the wound for you, the nurse, to bind?
  The war is over . . . 20 years past.
  No more horror . . . no more terror.
  Back in the States. Back to safety and security.

Where is the Pain? 'Big boys don't cry' you know.
Fear?
Being strong and fearless are what makes 'a few good *MEN*'. . . right?"
My deeper self knew what it had experienced and could not be convinced:
"Feelings *are*.
They have an energy that is real . . . whether we acknowledge them
    . . . or not.
Anger . . . fear . . . pain . . . guilt . . . helplessness . . . loneliness . . .
    uncertainty
They're like orphans no one wants . . .
They lurk . . . haunt . . . betray . . . smother . . .
Soldiers wall them off as fast as they can . . . "
My shallower selves were still not deterred:
"Embracing negative feelings only makes soldiers feel bad . . .
What's wrong with walling them off . . . behind hardened stoicism . . .
        into unconsciousness . . .
    where soldiers don't have to look at them . . .
        or feel them . . .
    . . . where they can't touch them . . .
        . . . where you don't have to fix them . . .
                    Do you?   Can you?"
My deeper self could now answer:
"I can't fix them . . .
    But I can be with them.
        My heart is willing to suffer   their sufferings.
I'm willing   to confront   the stoic wall
                    they hide behind.
        I'm willing to learn how to
                walk in the woods
                    with the wounded warrior.

Recovering from War: Poems by Women who Served in Vietnam[1]

The Best Act in Pleiku.
No One under 18 Admitted
(by Sharon Grant)
I kissed a Negro, trying to breathe life into him.
When I was a child—back in the world—

the drinking fountains said, "White Only."
His cold mouth tasted of dirt and marijuana.
He died and I put away the things of a child.

Do You Really Want to Know
(by Bobbie Trotter)
 Do you really want to know
 how you can help me?
Then don't turn your back on me
as if I was to blame!
You share in this too.
I did the dirty work,
the least you can do
is listen to me.

At Peace
(by Lily Lee Adams)
Now I feel at peace with myself
All the anger has left
It was the sediment
At the bottom of the bottle
That I couldn't reach
But I finally got it out.

"Thanks Nurse"
(by Diane Carlson Evans)
I am as much with the
Dead as with the living.
Facing the wall, I encounter something
I left behind so many
Years ago.
I am lifted away
And reunited with those who suffered
And died and left me
Alone.
Left me alone with the memories of them.
And left me too numb to cry.
As I put my hands on the hard granite

and touched the names of those who
Died, 1968-'69, I no longer
Felt alone.
Those who had died, came back
at that moment,
Allowed me to grieve, embraced me
And touched a part of my
Soul I had thought was gone.
That vague place in my Life,
Vietnam, which could not bring forth
Emotion or feelings
Or tears.
It was such a relief to cry now, to
feel again. It was so strange.
I felt unbearable sadness, and yet
Set free—free of an intangible
Burden.

Creating Safe Emotional Spaces

This appendix provides my suggestions for creating a safe emotional space with veterans. I try to help them feel comfortable while emerging emotionally *if they so choose*. I can do damage if I push. I also do damage by not asking difficult questions. My job is to open the door without pushing.

I try to be provocative with my questions and, at the same time, create safety for them to answer honestly or not answer at all, communicating that I respect whatever choice he/she makes. Thus, I often ask a difficult question and then sit quietly. It is the silence that is the most important part of the intervention. Sometimes the silence creates some anxiety; it is the anxiety that often takes them deeper into themselves and keeps the dialogue from being superficial or purely social.

Before Interventions Can Begin: Self-Awareness

Before any interventions will be effective, I have to honestly confront my own judgmental attitudes toward veterans, recognizing the value and meaning that military influences have on veterans' lives and deaths, and *want* to hear and serve veterans. This attitude fosters trust and diminishes phoniness. Gaining trust is essential in creating a safe emotional environment. It often must be done quickly because the dying person may only have a few hours or days to build a relationship. Becoming trustworthy is how trust is gained. Learning how to touch my own anger, fear, pain, guilt, loneliness, helplessness, and stoicism provides the foundation. This process requires a personal willingness to be vulnerable. (See Chapter 2 for my own self-awareness journey.)

Language That Creates Space

Developing the courage to be completely honest in communication, while simultaneously giving patients enough room to maintain full control also builds trust. Any pushing or imposing personal views or judgments can create barriers. I've learned to speak honestly and directly. At the same time, I provide ambiguous modifiers (like "probably," "maybe," "might," "sometimes," "usually," "a bit," "sort of," "I wonder") to give the patient room and control to direct or redirect dialogue if I'm going in the wrong direction or if I have assessed needs inaccurately. This language also conveys my understanding that I don't know the answers, and that the patient has abilities to figure it out. At the same time, it allows me to bring my ideas and experiences in the open for their consideration. (Note usage of ambiguous modifiers in sections that follow).

"Image" Words Create Space

"Image" words and metaphors are especially powerful. I incorporate them into dialogue because they have unique relevant meanings that access their unconscious (See Chapter 7).

When a patient speaks about feeling "trapped," "lost," "reeling," "pulled in every direction," "paralyzed," or "wilted"—images appear in my mind. I reference their image words intermittently in our conversation. "You told me you feel like you're *trapped* between a rock and a hard place. Tell me what that feels like." Later, I might ask, "Tell me what you think might give you some breathing space between that rock and hard place" or "How can I help make that hard place a bit softer today?"

Veterans often use battle metaphors to describe their relationship with death. I try to modify their metaphor: "Fighting attitudes were important on the battlefield, but you're not on a battlefield now. It's okay to surrender, to let go, so you can have a peaceful relationship with death," or "I know the last time you experienced death was on a battlefield. Death was probably ugly and violent then, but you're not on a battlefield now. Most people have very peaceful deaths. It's okay to relax and open up to death."

Interrupting

For interactions to be therapeutic, it is sometimes necessary to direct or redirect dialogue. This approach is not being rude; it's the reality of limited time. It's also necessary if dialogue is going to be elevated from a social interaction to a therapeutic interaction. "I'd like to hear more about this, but my time is limited. Tell me more about _____," or "I'm sorry to interrupt, but I needed to know more about _____."

Validating Suffering

Validating suffering is one of the most important contributions I can make
to the veteran's healing process; it helps both of us acknowledge that there's
a problem, which is not always easy for people who are stoic. Validating suffering is a willingness to acknowledge and bear witness to patients' difficult
experiences. It means resisting the urge to tell them, "It'll get better," "Count
your blessings," "Don't be so negative," or any of the other things that indi-
rectly communicate, "Don't tell me your problems. Don't let yourself feel
human. Put up that stoic wall and hide behind it."

Veterans often bear heavy sufferings, especially at the end of life.
Platitudes about smiling or keeping their chins up are just another way of
telling them to hide behind a stoic wall. Saying these kinds of things can also
erode their self-confidence. One patient told me, "I'm scared and miserable,
but everyone keeps telling me things are going to get better. I must be weak,
or I wouldn't feel so bad." We sell people short when we don't respect their
capacity to suffer. We miss the opportunity to affirm their courage in carrying their load.

Simple statements that affirm their suffering can have the opposite
effect. Statements such as "You've had a hard go of it" or "It takes a lot to go
through all of this" tell the patients that someone understands how difficult
their situation is. Patients have told me how grateful they are for these statements because it lessens their sense of isolation.

Asking About Military History

Many veterans don't call themselves veterans. They reserve that title for those
veterans who are service-connected for injuries or who have been in combat.
If asked if they are a veteran, they might reply, "No." Instead, ask if they have
served in the military.

Don't assume all noncombat veterans did not sustain trauma. Many
served in dangerous assignments. Rather than asking a veteran if they are a
combat vet, ask them if they've served in a "dangerous duty assignment."

When assessing military history, don't assume all combat veterans sustained trauma; some had "safe" assignments. Don't assume that those who
sustained trauma have PTSD; most do not. Our job is to carefully and
respectfully open the door inviting stories of trauma to come forth. Our job
is never to force stories; forcing can cause damage. Our job is to open the

door without pushing.

Ask open-ended questions that give the veteran control over how much or how little they choose to reveal. How the question is asked is more important than what is asked because it reveals your intent. I will often ask generalized questions such as: "Tell me a little bit about how things went for you in the military," or "How did your experiences in the military mold and shape your life?"

Confronting Stoicism

Stoicism is important, even essential, especially on a battlefield. It creates protection from untrustworthy influences. It's the *relationship* to stoicism that might need modification. It can be used inappropriately to block energy and emotion from self or interfere with expressing love to others. Stoicism can also contribute to veterans' underreporting their fear, emotional pain, and physical pain. I try to open the door for them to consider alternatives. "I know a lot of veterans put on a macho front and don't want to take pain medication, but pain can consume your energy. You need your energy for other things now."

I also have come to believe that the building blocks of stoic walls are pride, control, and independence. In my early career, I often dealt with pride by helping veterans "save face." I would also agree with patients that "things will get better," colluding with the illusion that health can return to normal even with death approaching. Now, I respond differently. I en-courage them to consider softening prideful ways so transitions can be navigated. I encourage them not to confuse stoicism with courage: "Anyone can hide behind a stoic wall of silence. It takes courage to reach out to connect with others or say 'I'm sorry' or 'I'm wrong'," or "You sound like a rather stubborn guy. Are you the kind of person who has a hard time compromising with others because when you do it feels like you're surrendering the battle or giving up?"

I also ask them to consider how pride might be affecting them: "Sounds like pride might be keeping you stuck, getting in the way of things going better for you," or "Most of us have a hard time owning our mistakes. Do you sometimes find it difficult to own your mistakes?"

My nursing training emphasized fostering control by giving patients choices, for example: "Do you want your medications with water or do you want juice?" "Do you want to get up now or later?" If patients complained about their confining world and how they had less control, I used to remind them of the choices and control they still had. Now, I give them choices, *and* I recognize the opportunity to penetrate stoicism by acknowledging their *lack* of control. I en-courage coming to peace with the helplessness by asking them to consider what they need to let go and what new things might they want to hold onto now that their situation has changed: "Your world has changed a lot. It's really shrinking," or "I find it hard to accept that some things are beyond my control. Tell me how *you're* doing with that."

Helplessness is often the feeling at the core of a strong need to control. I try to help them encounter their helplessness: "It can be hard to wait for death to come, to know it's not on your timetable," or "It's tough to realize we can't control the world, that we're not God." Helping them recognize the relationship between anger and helplessness can be beneficial: "Sometimes veterans tell me feeling helpless makes them angry. I imagine it's hard for a soldier to learn how to surrender, to let go."

I don't try to affirm their self-sufficiency anymore. It only reinforces independence they no longer have as they are dying. Instead, I validate their suffering and en-courage reckoning: "It's hard to not be able to do things for yourself any more," or "It's not easy to be at the mercy of others now." I try to guide them into taking responsibility for their needs and asking for help: "Some veterans tell me asking for help is humiliating. Tell me how helplessness makes *you* feel," or "Are you the kind of person who can accept things are changing and ask for help, or do you sometime try to pretend nothing has changed and things can go back to the way they used to be?"

Affirming Qualities that Promote Healing: Honesty, Humility, Courage

I try to counteract pride, independence, and control by helping veterans value qualities they have that will transform stoicism: "It takes a lot of courage to open yourself to your emotions and fears. I admire that," and "I appreciate your honesty, with yourself and with me. It's refreshing," and "You're accepting life on its own terms now rather than trying to impose your own. It's a humbling process. Humility is a *good* thing, an honorable quality I see in you."

Affirming and Validating Feelings

Veterans can often talk about their feelings; they have a more difficult time feeling their feelings. Compartmentalizing feelings can sometimes lock up vitality and interfere with healing; it traps energy. I try to give them permission to feel:

> "I know it can be hard for men to express their feelings, but now may not be a time to pretend like nothing is going on, that nothing has changed."
>
> "It may be difficult to express the hurt you might be feeling. It may be tempting to try to hide it and act like everything is going on like normal. It takes a lot of energy to pretend."
>
> "Now is a time when you might want to consider letting yourself be honest with yourself, and maybe with a few others too."
>
> "Are you willing to own your _____ (pain, fear, guilt, anger, loneliness, helplessness, etc.)?"
>
> "There's no shame in feeling your feelings. Feelings have vitality. They're meant to be shared with those who love you. It's okay to recognize your needs and ask for help when you need it."
>
> "How's your heart today, your inward heart?"
>
> "I can see you are comfortable talking about the _____ (hurt, anger, guilt, helplessness, etc.)? I'm wondering if there are times when you let yourself *feel* your _____ (hurt, anger, guilt, helplessness), when you let the feelings move down from your head to your heart?"
>
> Empowering silent voices: "If your _____ (anger, fear, cancer, liver, Deeper Self) could speak, what might it say?"
>
> "I know you said you feel "fine;" but you don't sound like you really mean it. I noticed you _____ (sighed, tightened up, seemed rather unconvinced, etc.) as you said it."
>
> Normalizing feelings conveys the naturalness and healthfulness of owning and expressing feelings: "Many veterans tell me they feel _____ (angry, scared, sad, guilty, helpless, lonely) when something like this happens." I also try to evaluate the intensity of their

feelings: "On a 0-10 scale, what number is your _____
(anger, guilt, pain, fear, helplessness)?" I don't try to
reduce that number. Instead, I ask them to tell me
what their (anger, guilt, pain, fear, helplessness) is
telling them. I don't try to lower a "10" feeling of helplessness by asking them what they can do to feel less
helpless. This attitude encourages them to hold onto
what is not holdable. Rather, I en-courage coming to
peace with the helplessness of dying by asking them to
consider what they need to let go and what new things
might they want to hold onto now that their situation
has changed.

Grief

Men often grieve differently than women. The goal is not to make them cry;
the goal is to help them grieve in whatever way they can. Sometimes actions,
such as planting a memorial tree, visiting the surviving family members, or
going to a gravesite may be more effective. However, it is still important to
give all grievers permission to cry, so they feel free to do so. Tears of sadness
contain stress chemicals that are not contained in tears of joy.[1]

"I see you choking down tears. I want you to know that it's okay to cry.
We say here that the only bad tears are uncried tears."

"It's good to see your tears; they're safe here."

"This is a very sad time. Tears are welcome here."

Guilt

Veterans often bear much guilt that can interfere with peace of mind and
peace of heart. ("If only I would have done _____, he'd still be here today. If
only . . . If only . . . If only . . . " "Why him and not me?") Guilt should lead
toward remorse and forgiveness. Guilt should teach, not punish. Sometimes
their guilt is irrational, and they think they are responsible for things over
which they had no control. (See Chapter 6 for details about guilt and forgiveness.)

I try to help patients sort through what they can learn from their guilt
so they can enter the work of forgiveness. There may also be irrational guilt
that they need to let go because they're trying to control something they had

no control over or they need to forgive themselves for not being God. (For example, they're not omniscient and omnipotent.) It's important that I orient myself to where a person is on the "disorders of responsibility spectrum" before I know what words to offer. For example, the last thing I want to tell someone who has a difficult time accepting responsibility is, "That's over. Let that go."

If they are responsible for harming others, a ritual of forgiveness can be developed to restore integrity (similar to the ritual for Paul in Chapter 5). Chaplains are another important resource. They are usually trained in both the process of forgiveness and the value of rituals.

Patients unwilling to assume little or any responsibility for a troubled relationship or situation: I try to help people appropriately assume some guilt. Instilling guilt can be threatening. I make sure I use plenty of ambiguous words (italics words in the quotes below) to give them plenty of room to accept, modify, or reject my offering. It also gives me room to be wrong if I've mis-assessed the situation. I've also learned to phrase questions in a way that educates patients on the value of guilt and how it can increase their power:

> "Some people *might* be tempted to think they have no role with trouble in a relationship. What are some of the *possible* ways you have succumbed to that temptation?"

> "Guilt can be an important teacher that leads toward healing and restoration. Can you tell me something about this situation in which you share *a little bit* of the guilt?"

> *Patients who assume too much guilt:* Some people have irrational guilt; it interferes with healing and recovery:

> "Are you thinking you're the only one who bears any responsibility in this situation? I'm *wondering* if you're able to let go of some things that *might not* be your responsibility."

> "I'm *wondering* what's making you think you're responsible for other people's feelings and actions?"

> "Sounds like you *might* be thinking you were psychic and could have foreseen the future so this could

have been prevented. Are you thinking you can be all
things to all people at all times—that you are omnipotent and omniscient—that you are God?"

"Are you willing to forgive yourself for not being
God? Are you willing to let yourself be human?"

Forgiveness

I usually encourage patients and family members to review their relationships
with honest self-appraisal, asking themselves some challenging questions:

"Is there anyone I harbor resentment toward?"

"Are there any relationships that are suffering
because I'm still holding onto hurt?"

"What relationships do I feel guilty about? Is the
guilt unreasonable and so I need to let it go? Is the guilt
reasonable prompting me to take an action to make
amends?"

"Do I need to forgive the world for being like it is?"

"Do I need to forgive God for not making the
world the way I want it?"

"What is keeping me from letting go?"

"What choices am I making to keep myself from
experiencing the healing power of forgiveness?"

"Am I willing to be free of resentment and blame?"

"Am I willing to stop being the victim?"

"What benefits are there for my allowing myself
to be the victim?"

"Am I willing to make a decision to forgive? On
a 0-10 scale, how willing am I to forgive?"

"Am I willing to do the work of forgiveness?"

I also help people accept apologies rather than rebuffing them with, "It's
okay. You don't need to apologize."

Encouraging People to Stay in the Struggle Required to Reckon with Suffering

Anxiety often surfaces as people confront difficult issues in their lives. We want to fight/flight the anxiety. Yet, it is often at this point that a break-through is about to happen. A shift in the relationship to the issue can then occur. I en-courage them to stay with the moment, to tolerate the anxiety: "What you're doing is hard. It's important," or "Stay with it. Answers may not come quickly, but when they do, they might be more satisfying," or "I'd encourage you to resist going for the quick fix or the easy way out. That may help you win the battle today but the war will still not be won."

Much of the work I do is simply supporting patient's feelings and struggles. Often that process is all that is required for the patient to come to peace with an issue with which he/she is struggling. Sometimes they require more; they require support for confronting the issue. When I'm assessing a patient's willingness to reckon with difficult issues, I'll often scale their will-ingness to change. Unlike words, intention will manifest itself in actions. So there's no point in helping someone reckon with something that they have no intention of changing: "On a 0-10 scale, how willing are you to change your relationship with this problem?" or "On a 0-10 scale, how willing are you to let go of _____ (bitterness, resentment, denial, resistance, etc.)?"

Author, Viktor Frankl emphasizes the need to change ourselves when we can't change a problem.[2] We have to change our *relationship to* the prob-lem; a shift in consciousness has to be made. I often ask questions that chal-lenge the relationship we maintain with our suffering.

"Tell me about the ways in which you have made the most out of this life situation? Tell me about the ways you have become bitter because of this?"

"Tell me about the ways you have used this disappointment as a cata-lyst for growth?" "Tell me about the ways that you have allowed this disap-pointment to cause you to never take risks again?"

"Tell me how this loss has caused you to make sure you learn how to connect with others in a meaningful way?" Tell me how this loss has given you the sense that the world owes you?"

Trauma: With or Without PTSD

Veterans who have served in dangerous duty assignments not only sustain physical injuries, they also sustain mental, emotional, social, spiritual, and moral injuries. In about 20%-30% of veterans, these injuries result in PTSD.[3]

It is the moral injury that often surfaces at end of life. The mental, social, and spiritual injuries sometimes interfere with their dealing with this moral injury. The symptoms of PTSD reflect many of the mental and emotional injuries. The social injuries often relate to difficulty fitting back into civilian culture and family. The spiritual injury might focus on how God could let war happen or question how God could allow such cruelty. The moral wound veterans sustain often relates to having had their pretrauma sense of what is right and wrong shattered. Their sense of what is fair and unfair is injured and needs healing.[4]

I usually ask an open-ended question when initially assessing trauma. Afterward, I sit quietly in silence for several seconds afterward, shifting into a low, quiet, abiding energy:

"You probably saw a lot of ugly things in that war. Is there anything that might still be troubling you now?"

"Many veterans who've not been in combat have sustained other kinds of trauma. Are there any traumas you've sustained that might still be troubling you a bit?"

I always validate their sufferings, whatever its source: physical, mental, emotional, social, spiritual, or moral.

"You've had to carry a lot of burdens. Fitting back into the world after war isn't easy."

"I would guess there have been times when you've been pretty angry at God for allowing the world to have war in it, for not intervening to protect people from cruelty."

"I would think the world was pretty confusing after you returned from war. All the rules had changed; much of what you were taught was violated."

Sometimes I express my speechlessness in response to the difficulties of someone's trials, uttering a low and respectful "WOW!" (**W**ith **O**ut **W**ords)

Many people surround the trauma imprint with a wall of silence. This wall needs to be respected; we should never force them to tell their stories. However, offering some quotes by other veterans may be able to give voice to their stories if they so choose. Then I sit silently. The story, lost in the soul, often comes to light with a simple nod of the head and a tear that escapes down the cheek. No words need be said. The tear tells the story; it is witnessed. Suffering is validated; healing begins:

"Sometimes, a vet will tell me he lost his soul in _____ (WWII, Korea, Vietnam, Iraq). Did something like that sort of happen with you?"

"Sometimes combat veterans tell me that when they killed others, they killed a part of themselves. Did you experience anything sort of like that?"

Families are also a source for veterans' experiences of war. A door can be opened by offering a quote heard by other family members:

"Some families have told me, 'Most of my brother remained in Vietnam.' Did anything like that sort of happen with your loved one?"

"Some family members have told me they didn't know the person who came back after the war, that their loved one was like a stranger, just a shell of the person they used to know. Have you experienced anything sort of like that with your loved one?"

Double Listening[5]

If the veteran feels guilty for causing trauma they didn't cause or couldn't control, I ask them how they got tricked into thinking they were responsible. Sometimes I ask how they've allowed trauma to take over their lives in an effort to determine if they are ready to reclaim their lives or determine what role irrational guilt is playing that keeps them holding onto it.

As I listen to stories of trauma, I also listen for stories of survival. It's a kind of double listening. No matter how victimized they've been, there are exceptions when they've transcended their suffering:

"Tell me about a time when you were able to stand up to blaming yourself."

I can be relentless in helping them discover this. I don't let people off the hook because I know that in some ways they've exerted enough power that provides enough hope to precipitate the conversation we are having. For example, one man told me he felt guilty even talking to me. Guilt often does that, reduces self-worth to disintegrated rubble. "So even though guilt told you not to come here, that you're not worth my time, you stood up to it? You told it you were coming here anyway. You told it you weren't going to listen to it?"

He nodded slightly, "I guess so."

"Good for you!" I high-fived him, sending him home with a homework assignment to strengthen his guilt-rebelling voice.

I also seek veteran's wisdom with questions such as:

"What have your sufferings taught you?"

"What would you teach others?"

"What wisdom do you have that might help me live my life better?"

Trauma With PTSD

Veterans may not even be aware of how their trauma history affected their current difficulties. Instead, they may feel worthless and filled with shame because they have been unable to live out their dreams. They might also associate death with horror, fear, and helplessness that they felt on the battlefield. They might fight death and need extra guidance in how to let go and "surrender."

The psychological aftermath of war sometimes leaves veterans thinking they are crazy: "You are not crazy. PTSD is a normal response to an abnormal situation. It was the situation that was crazy. If you weren't affected by the war, then you might be crazy."

I often urge them to seek information and support at a *Vet Center*. *Vet Centers* have been established around the country by veterans to help veterans come home from war. *Vet Centers* are usually not associated with VAs and are therefore sometimes more trusted by veterans. A veteran doesn't have to be enrolled in the VA system to access *Vet Centers*.

Flashbacks are normal as the mind tries to reckon with what has happened. When traumatic images surface, I en-courage veterans to give the images voice so feelings have a mode of expression. Oftentimes the images will soften and change. Trauma internalized can make people think they are the problem. Externalizing the trauma helps them understand they have a problem. Giving voice to trauma helps them gather scattered pieces of broken self, reowning exiled fragments.[6]

Some clinicians may find it helpful to screen for PTSD. A formalized instrument asks the following questions: "In your life, have you ever had any experience that was so frightening, horrible, or upsetting that, in the past month, you:
   • Have had nightmares about it or thought about it when you did not want to?
   • Tried hard not to think about it or went out of your way to avoid situations that reminded you of it?
   • Were constantly on guard, watchful, or easily startled?
   • Felt numb or detached from others, activities, or your surroundings?"
Answering "yes" to two or more questions suggests need for further evaluation.[7]

Assessing Dying Veterans' Needs

When admitting patients for end-of-life care or doing consults for emotional support, I have a blueprint that elicits three perspectives from the patient:

- A sense of their *past* story, including how the military might have impacted them.
- Their *current* relationship to the dilemma they are facing with poor health, including their identification of their most pressing need.
- Their hopes for the *future*, including what they need so they can "die healed."

En-couraging Preparation for Death: Seven Steps of Living and Dying Healed

The seven steps of peaceful living and dying are essential, forming the core practice for helping people live their deaths:[8]

"You may be wondering about what you can do to prepare for your death; what you can do so you have a 'good' death, die with peace. There are seven things you can do to die healed." We talk about what "dying healed" means. I give them considerations for reflection: "All of us have done things to hurt each other; none of us are saints. Now is a time to reflect on people you may have hurt and consider asking for forgiveness. Think about those who have hurt you, as well as any hurts you may be holding onto. Consider letting them go, offering forgiveness. Think about who in your circle of friends and family may benefit from an expression of your love. Think about those people who have impacted your life. Who might benefit from an expression of gratitude for having touched your life?" I encourage them to be as specific as they can in these contemplations and also affirm they need not do this with me, but privately.

Then I inform them about the last steps: "The next thing is the hardest but probably the most important and that is to say goodbye: to all those you love and want to hold onto, to say goodbye to this world and everything in it; to say goodbye to all that's been the same. Let yourself grieve. After you've done these five steps, then your new job is to relax and let go of all that is familiar so you can be free, to open up to all that is new and different coming your way."

I en-courage family members to do the process with their dying loved one too.

I affirm the difficulty of the process: "I'm making it sound easy. It's not. It takes honesty. It takes courage. It takes humility." I highlight the value of the process for myself: "I do this process myself at the end of each day. It's a good method for living healed."

Helping Patients Encounter Difficult Subjects like Death

I strive to be completely honest in my communication, while simultaneously giving them enough room to maintain full control. Any pushing or imposing personal views or judgments can add blocks to the wall. I speak honestly and directly. I try to maintain a tension between direct honesty and ambiguous fluidity:

"All of us need to be prepared for death so that when it happens nothing is left unsaid or undone. Whether you die today or 10 years from now, it's good to be prepared."

"If you died today, what would be left unsaid or undone?"

"What do you need to do to get ready for your death?"

"We can't control the quantity of your life, but we can help control the quality . . . "

"I'm sorry this has happened to you."

"Pretend like you knew you were going to die today. What hopes would you have?"

"What is your idea of a peaceful death?"

"We CAN help. I'm here to give you options."

Interventions for Community Agencies or Partnerships

Eliminate as many "triggers" for PTSD as possible. Remember that coming into a hospital (especially a VA hospital) can trigger past military memories of barracks, procedures, unsafe environments, past combat hospitalizations, visiting injured comrades, etc. A government hospital and its employees may not be trusted by Vietnam vets. On the other hand, a VA might be a source of comfort, belonging, security, and camaraderie.

Loud or unexpected sounds will startle people with PTSD. Don't touch them without first calling out their name or letting them see you.

No bed alarms for veterans with PTSD.

No restraints or confinements for veterans who were former POWs. Even tight bed clothes or bed linens can trigger memories of being imprisoned.

Express appreciation to all veterans for service to our country.

Provide symbols of appreciation for service to our country: certificates, pins, cards, handshakes accompanied by personal expressions of gratitude.

Acknowledge to the family the hardship the military experience might have had on their lives. Provide symbols to them for their sacrifices made to support the veteran.

Distinguish between "terminal restlessness," delirium, and PTSD. Know that some of the medications used for terminal restlessness may be ineffective for PTSD.

Before medicating agitation, determine its source because pain, full or infected bladders, constipation, low oxygen levels, PTSD, medication interactions, and terminal restlessness can cause agitation. The treatment is different for each. Our Hospice performs a "7 P Assessment" for agitation: pain, pee, poop, pulse ox, PTSD, polypharmacy, and pre-Hospice. Though it may sound crass, it's effective.

Remember that some of the usual treatments for PTSD may not be practical in the last few days of life because the conscious mind is weakening. For some, grounding in reality is not feasible; instead, enter the metaphor or hallucination with them. Provide them with whatever they need to feel safe. Safety is always the essential ingredient.

Encourage therapeutic rituals for integrating past trauma and providing hope for the future (See Chapter 5 and Appendices E and F).

Veterans and their families may have bereavement needs that require special consideration (See Appendix D).

Help veterans to know about the law that requires VAs to provide hospice care or purchase it for all enrolled veterans *regardless of category*.[9]

Require all staff to watch the DVD "Wounded Warriors: Their Last Battle," and use the follow-up video to provide training. Contact the author through the publisher for copies.

Consider this book as required reading for staff.

Have all staff read the NHPCO and VA monograph, *VA Transforms End of Life Care,* available online at: www.NHPCO.org/veterans. Scroll down to "Helpful Resources." Click on "VA Transforms End-of-Life Care for Veterans."

Consult the Hospice-Veterans Partnership toolkit for relevant resources: vha08spt1/sites/pallcare/default.aspx.

Modify admission forms to include questions about veteran status and combat/trauma history.

Inform all veterans of their eligibility for free burial in a National Cemetery. Let them know that spouses are eligible for burial there as well.

For cemeteries in your vicinity, see www.cem.va.gov.

Consider assigning veteran volunteers to veteran patients.

Consider transporting patients to the morgue or funeral home under an American flag quilt.

If you have an inpatient hospice facility, consider decorating one wing with military décor or symbols and place veterans there.

When admitting to an inpatient facility, consider placing patients in a two-patient room with another veteran. The camaraderie is often mutually supportive.

Feature articles about veterans or veteran volunteers in newsletters.

Consider participating in the NHPCO and National VA Hospice Veteran partnership. Contact NHPCO or Department of Veterans Affairs for information.

Consider forming an "emergency support team" with your local *Vet Center* that can respond to traumatic experiences that might surface at end of life. Remember that veterans do not have to be enrolled in a VA in order to access *Vet Centers* and that *Vet Center* staff visit veterans in their homes.

Consider working with the VA in your community and the *Vet Center* to provide bereavement care for families of veterans returning from Iraq and Afghanistan.

Support or provide ceremonies of recognition for Memorial Day, July 4, Veterans Day.

Consult Tidewell Hospice at www.tidewell.org for information about providing counseling for: families in the military, families caring for veterans, and bereavement for families of veterans.

Appendix C

Posttraumatic Stress Disorder (PTSD)

This appendix provides more detailed information about PTSD. My curiosity about PTSD was stimulated because I wanted to better understand the impact that combat experiences made on my patients. Thus, when I went to graduate school to become a Nurse Practitioner, I decided to focus on psychiatric nursing. The *Diagnostic and Statistical Manual of Mental Disorders* (DSM) was the fundamental reference for the courses I took. Used as the handbook for defining mental health, the DSM identifies characteristics for each mental disorder. I wasted no time looking up Posttraumatic Stress Disorder (PTSD) in the DSM.[1] I read about the six criteria that must be present for the diagnosis:

- Exposure to a traumatic event experienced with fear, helplessness, or horror
- The traumatic event is persistently reexperienced through one or more of the following symptoms:
  - Recollections
  - Dreams
  - Flashbacks, hallucinations, or illusions
  - Distress at cues that symbolize the trauma
  - Physiologic responses when confronted with cues reminiscent of the trauma
- Avoidance behaviors and emotional numbing exhibited by three or more of the following:
  - Avoidance of thoughts, feelings, or conversations related to the trauma
  - Avoidance of activities, places, or people that arouse recollection
  - Inability to recall certain critical aspects of the trauma
  - Lack of interest in significant activities formerly enjoyed
  - Feelings of detachment or emotional distancing from others
  - Restricted range of affect (limited emotional expression)
  - Sense of a foreshortened future (inability to accomplish cherished life goals)
- Persistent symptoms of increased arousal manifested by two or more

symptoms that include:
- Difficult sleep patterns
- Irritability or outbursts of anger
- Difficulty concentrating
- Hypervigilance (staying on guard and unable to calm down or relax)
- Exaggerated startle response to noises, being touched, etc.
• Symptoms persist for at least one month
• The disturbance of symptoms causes significant distress or impairment

Because PTSD had only recently been added to the DSM, I assumed it was a new disorder. Then one day, I heard a sermon about Job, a man in the Old Testament; I was intrigued enough to read more about him in the Bible. When I did, I realized I was reading a description of PTSD centuries before it was given a name. After experiencing the deaths of his 10 children, failing health, and the loss of his wealth, Job understandably became angry with God, questioning what he had done to deserve his fate. Job thinks he can gain reprieve from his torment while he's asleep, but he's wrong. He graphically describes the nightmares of PTSD: "My bed shall comfort me, my couch shall ease my complaint. Then, God, you affright me with dreams and visions terrify me, so that *I should prefer choking and death rather than my pains.*"[2]

Though its victims preferred choking and death over the affliction, PTSD was not included in the psychiatric disorders curriculum at my university. My graduate school professor told me PTSD was not important for us to learn since most students didn't work with veterans. I reminded her that PTSD was not a uniquely military experience. "Victims of crime, abuse, natural disasters, and violence commonly experience PTSD," I told her. "Even policemen, ambulance drivers, and trauma counselors experience what is called 'vicarious trauma'." I added that the bereavement literature identifies complicated grief as PTSD.

My pleas fell on deaf ears. My professor said PTSD had only recently been recognized by the psychiatric community. I resisted the urge to read the Bible to her, and kept it in military terms. "But that doesn't mean it wasn't around. It just means we didn't recognize it. Civil War soldiers called it 'soldier's heart,' World War I soldiers called it 'shell shock' or 'battle fatigue'."

She remained unconvinced. I did gain consent from a different professor in another course to focus on PTSD for a group assignment. Three of us who worked for the VA provided a classroom dramatization reflecting a composite experience of the suffering we often witnessed with our combat veterans. Afterward, one pensive student responded, "My boyfriend was killed in Vietnam. I've never gotten over it. Now that I realize how PTSD might have affected his life, maybe death wasn't the worst outcome he could have suffered."

When my classmate said this, I thought about some of the things I'd heard my patients say that made me think she might be right. "Ninety percent of me died in that war" or "I lost my soul in that war," are statements I've sometimes heard.

Often veterans speak of survivor's guilt. "If only I would have done _____, he'd still be here today. It should have been me who died."

As often as not, however, silence about war experiences enshrouds PTSD. While they were in the military, they kept silent because of the attached stigma and loss of promotion opportunities if anyone knew they had PTSD. After discharge from service, their silence was often a way to protect their families from the trauma they experienced. Others kept silent because "it's impossible to explain; no one who hasn't been there can understand what it's like." Some weren't allowed to talk about it; they were on secret missions and signed a contract stating they wouldn't divulge their experiences. Some have said they kept quiet because when they did speak up "I wasn't believed;" this attitude only added insult to injury. Many veterans don't talk about their experiences because they don't know who they can trust with their stories; many people don't want to hear about the ugly things they saw or did.

Whether they speak about it or not, an expression in their eyes gives it away, a kind of deadness as they detach from themselves or others. Dissociation from feelings is often the only way they can get through horror. The DSM describes this as "psychic numbing" or "emotional anesthesia." Coupled with military training that taught them stoicism, this numbness can leave veterans isolated physically, mentally, emotionally, and spiritually. Isolation is a common way for traumatized veterans to deal with their experiences. This can cause serious impairments of emotional intimacy in relationships.

Alcohol abuse can cause further detachment for some veterans. Alcohol usage was encouraged in military service. It was easily available and accessible in places on base without under-age limitations. It was a convenient way to numb feelings of loneliness when away from home. It shouldn't be surprising that soldiers excessively used alcohol or drugs after discharge from military service to "flight" unwanted feelings stuck behind stoic walls or to numb traumatic war memories. On the other hand, drinking sometimes allows hidden stories to surface, though it often accomplishes little. Poignantly, a veteran's daughter told me, "He only wanted to tell his war stories when he was drinking, but when he was drinking, we didn't want to be around him."

Despite veterans' best efforts to remain disconnected from their trauma, there are times when their walled-off self emerges anyway. When it does, it sometimes comes out angrily, like hurled grenades. With traumatic memories intruding and interrupting, it's not surprising that people with PTSD might struggle with irritability and anger. Driving habits might become reckless; career patterns might disintegrate into job-hopping. Frustrations, disagreements, or disappointments incite aggression; anger often masks pain.

In this state, veterans can overreact to otherwise innocuous stimuli. A car backfires triggering a veteran with PTSD to "hit the deck." A helicopter flies overhead and a Vietnam veteran seeks cover. A balloon pops at a birthday party and a veteran with PTSD decides he won't go to parties again. A veteran, ambushed in the woods or jungle, no longer enjoys wooded environments. Rain triggers memories of monsoons. Hunting takes on new, no-longer-enjoyable meanings. Open fields (that made combat veterans vulnerable to attack) mean inability to enjoy the expanse of open areas anymore. If a vet experienced a bridge blowing up, he may no longer be able to drive over bridges, altering driving patterns extensively. News reports of current wars or mass traumas trigger memories. If children were crying when a village was invaded, a child's cry now, even their own child's, sets off panic and anger.

I've seen how sounds or suspicious actions precipitate hypervigilance (staying on guard) because trust in the world has been violated and adrenalin stays on call for rescue from the next threat. I've heard accounts of veterans repeatedly getting up through the night to look out the windows to assure themselves that no enemy threats lurk in their civilian neighborhoods. In restaurants, they find a seat against the wall to make sure that nothing is behind their back and that they are in position to survey the environment. Hypervigilant behaviors can become extreme, developing into paranoia. Paranoia helps save lives in combat zones, but it can destroy personal relationships.

One of my patients had been a World War II prisoner-of-war (POW). He became extremely agitated with flashbacks of the POW camp; he believed he was actually there. We treated him with high doses of sedatives and provided one-on-one nursing care, but nothing seemed to help. Though the patient had been urinating regularly, one of the nurses checked to see if the patient's bladder was emptying incompletely because full bladders can cause agitation. A bladder scan revealed four times the normal amount of urine. We inserted a urinary catheter; he immediately calmed down and returned from the POW camp. It was a graphic reminder that any noxious stimuli (like a full bladder) can trigger noxious combat memories.

Not surprisingly, PTSD often surfaces at night. Nightmares have freedom to rise from unconsciousness. The kind of nightmares my patients describe are unlike any I've ever had. They are anguishing nightmares that wreak havoc to rest and slumber. Many wives of patients have told me about trying to awaken their husband to rescue him from torment only to be mistaken for the enemy and then to be struck or restrained. Many people with PTSD become unable to fall to sleep, knowing these nightmares are awaiting them.

In my work at the VA, I've seen that some veterans with PTSD seem to age prematurely. Often they look 10 years older than they are. With the adrenalin of the autonomic nervous system turned to the "on" position much of the time and the restorative power of sleep interrupted with nightmares, this phenomenon is not surprising.

Aging and illness, in general, can make it more difficult to reckon with PTSD. Likewise, PTSD can be exacerbated by aging and illness. Memories can no longer be suppressed so easily. More than one veteran's wife has told me, "He's talked about that war more in the last year than he has in all the previous years put together." Even veterans' end-of-life experience can be influenced by their previous exposure to death. They sometimes come to our Hospice unit associating death with the fear, horror, and helplessness that they had experienced on the battlefield. This fear adds yet another layer of complexity to their end-of-life care. When I try to tell them how peaceful death can be, they don't believe it.

The DSM states that the severity, duration, and proximity of an individual's exposure to a traumatic event are the most important factors influencing the likelihood of developing PTSD. Most references cite PTSD incidence among veterans to be around 20%-30%[3] depending on which war they fought in, the branch of service they were in, their role in the war, and other factors. The silence that surrounds PTSD, no doubt, causes underreporting, suggesting that the incidence may be even higher.[4]

Ground troops in face-to-face combat who see the results of their killing are at higher risk than those whose roles distance them from the carnage. For example infantry soldiers are more susceptible to PTSD than pilots; Army and Marine Corps divisions are more susceptible than Air Force or Navy.[5] As one patient told me, "The people I killed with my bayonet are the ones I can't forget. The killing is much more personal." I've heard similar comments from snipers who saw the result of their killing up close through their rifle scopes.

Some sources say that the act of killing is the single most important factor generating PTSD.[6,7,8] It is this moral injury that soldiers sustain that I sometimes see surface as they face their deaths years later. Experiencing or witnessing violence can cause PTSD in anyone; but the difference with veterans is that they committed much of the violence. This is a deeper level of traumatization.[9]

The DSM cites other factors that increase risk of PTSD. These include lack of social supports, family history, childhood experiences, personality variables, and preexisting mental disorders. It also notes the condition can develop "without any predisposing conditions."[10]

When I do presentations about veterans, I set the tone by playing a recording of war sounds. Inevitably, the audience becomes irritated and asks me to turn it off. "These sounds mean nothing to us except that they are disrupting our safe, comfortable environment," I tell them. "Imagine if you were in combat. These sounds would mean that death is coming. How would we feel then?"

I don't know if any of us, who have not experienced war, can fully appreciate its impact. The closest I can imagine is the terrorist attack on the World Trade Center and Pentagon on 9/11 2001. I remember how our whole world stopped. Our lives were suspended as we sat on edge to learn our fate. I think about what it might have been if there had been a 9/12 with the Empire State building bombed or a 9/13 with the White House burned. Maybe there's not a 9/14, but we didn't know that, and so we stayed on guard. Meanwhile, the media are saying: "We don't know where the terrorists are, but we know they're in your neighborhood." It's hard to imagine how we would live day after day under these kinds of circumstances. One thing I do know: there would be a greater appreciation for PTSD because a lot of us would have it.

Other Ramifications of PTSD That Are NOT Listed in the DSM

The DSM does not identify anger, resentment, fear, guilt, and shame as an aftereffect of trauma, but it's a theme I sometimes observe. It causes suffering and undermines veterans' goals, even if they don't realize they have PTSD. "I came back from the war and enrolled in college, but I just couldn't seem to focus. I wasn't so sure of my goals anymore," more than one veteran has told me.

Relationships sometimes suffer. "I can't believe how I treated my first wife," different veterans have said. "I don't know what got into me." Family life can be affected. "All I ever wanted was a family, yet the kids got on my nerves, and all I seemed to do was yell. They were scared of me." Another veteran added, "I tried to run my family like a minimilitary unit. It didn't work too well." Sometimes the could-have-been future relationships were not to be. Several veterans have told me they never married because they knew they couldn't be good spouses or parents.

Young people 18, 19, and 20 years old often naively think they will give their three or four years to their country to fight a war and then resume their lives unaffected when discharged. In fact, the American public expects them to do that. Guilt and a sense of inadequacy heighten as hopes are dashed or dreams are unable to be achieved in the way society, parents, or the veteran himself had planned. Shame is often a common denominator; they feel like they let others down or could have done better. The self-hate this sometimes generates can result in either fear and isolation or anger and violence. Furthermore, there's often a lack of awareness about how failure to achieve hopes might relate to combat exposure. I've seen this kind of guilt as veterans near the end of their lives. I call it the guilt of unfulfilled longings for the life not lived.

Appendix D

Family and Bereavement Considerations[1]

The military culture can also impact bereavement for veterans and their family members.[2] This appendix will highlight some of the issues that require consideration when responding to the grief of both veterans and their families. Veterans and their families are susceptible to experiencing complicated grief. Complicated grief is PTSD: the surviving family member repeatedly experiences their loved one's death, tries to avoid or detach from triggers that cause reminders of the loss, and experiences intrusive memories that cause anxiety, anger, or grief.

First, I'll identify issues for family members. In one way or another, the soldier changes after war and their relationships with others can never be the same. Much of a family's suffering surrounds grieving the loss these changes cause. Helping families come to peace with their changed loved one usually involves helping them grieve so they can let go of how their prewar family member was and open up to a new relationship that includes the changes that their relationship incurs. It means letting go of old expectations and exploring ways to birth new expectations within relationships.

Stoicism can affect whole family systems. Grief might be hidden by a silent or angry façade. If the veteran was "career military," the family may have lived in numerous places for short periods of time. This situation can have different effects on bereavement. Because they have not established roots, there may not be a network of support that facilitates effective grieving. On the other hand, because of their frequent moving, families of veterans may readily reach out for support because they've learned how to ask for help and form new bonds quickly.

If the veteran had PTSD, especially if it became exacerbated during their dying process, the family caregivers may be exhausted and not have the energy required for grieving. They may have become so consumed with caregiving that they lost their own life or sense of self, which makes recovery from grief more difficult. When this kind of difficulty occurs, we provide caregiver kits to acknowledge the struggle of family and friends to provide care to patients. The "care bag" was designed by one of the nurses, Susan Schaeffer. It contains symbolic reminders: a rubber band "to remind you to be flexible because things might not go the way you want," a band-aid "to heal hurt feelings," a pencil "to list your feelings," an eraser to "remind you that everyone makes mistakes and that's okay," gum "to chew sticky stuff when you feel you're falling apart," a tea bag "to help you relax daily and take time for yourself," a bell "to remind you to let others know what you need," and tissue because "it's okay to cry." When caregivers receive these "gifts," they often respond with tears. Frequently forgotten, consumed with demands, the ritualized gesture validates caregivers' suffering and encourages personal needs. We are also careful to not give them to caregivers who were reluctant to caregive because they were too self-absorbed.

Because family members are often "unsung heroes," we provide a pin of an angel with an American flag as a dress to family members to acknowledge the sacrifices they have made for our country and its veterans. We don't do this routinely with all family members, lest it becomes rote. Rather, we ceremonially pin them when we hear how the military impacted them or their loved one. In this way, the pin can have profound meaning.

If PTSD is identified for the first time as a veteran is dying, the impact on family needs to be factored into their bereavement needs. Some feel relief saying, "I'm so glad to know it has a name. I knew something was wrong, but I didn't know what. Now this makes sense." Others might feel guilty. "I wish I would've realized this sooner, I would have _____ (listened more carefully, gotten him help, been more patient and understanding, etc.)"

Family members may need help in understanding that a veteran's inability to grieve someone's death might be due to their fear of unresolved grief from comrades who died in combat. This fear can sometimes cause the veteran to detach from his grief; otherwise "If I start crying, I'll never be able to stop."

Family members might have anger or bitterness about their veteran not getting a medal, service-connected disability, or pension. These feelings can interfere with effective grieving.

Family members, who are receiving a military-related pension that ceases upon the veteran's death, may seek to keep the veteran alive for financial gain, seeking futile treatments that interfere with peaceful dying and effective bereavement processes.

One of my hopes is that community hospices will start partnering with the VA in their communities and the *Vet Centers* to provide bereavement care for families of soldiers dying in Iraq and Afghanistan. Tidewell Hospice in Sarasota, Florida is already doing this. Additionally, they provide support groups for military families who have loved ones in a combat theatre.[3]

Ben was a friend of mine who was a World War II veteran. Over time, I came to see how stoicism and his combat experiences had impacted his life. When Ben died, I met his five adult children, all of whom lived out of state. I could see that some of them felt distant from their father. I wrote them a letter to offer insight that might provide a healing perspective for how the effects of the military had impacted them. Later, I learned from Ben's wife that this letter helped their children to better understand their father. It also helped one daughter to stop blaming herself for her father's cold treatment in her childhood. This is the letter:

> Dear Susan, Greg, Jane, Paul, and Amy,
>
> As I came away from the funeral service last night, I was left with a desire to share my own story about your Dad. I have known your Dad for the past 10 years as part of our church community. He started a small group in his home, and we have been meeting monthly since that time. Your Dad was careful to say in the first meeting that this would not be the kind of meeting where people "spill their guts," and your Dad kept his word about that for five years. One night, however, your Dad started talking about the death of your sister. As he spoke, it became apparent that the death of this daughter at age five had been deeply disturbing, though he had never let himself grieve. Instead, he had boxed up his pain, hoping it would go away. Now, 40 years later, here it was again. This time though, he let himself feel his pain. He told of his despair over losing a child at that tender age, and he let himself cry. He was embarrassed at first, but soon the emotion gave way to the sobs of tears he had held back so long. Your Mom said it was the first time she'd ever seen him cry. I think your Dad was a little different after that day. A part of his heart was unlocked and his sharing became more open, his feelings expressed more freely.
>
> I also think of your Dad at our 4th of July party. We did a tribute to the veterans for the freedom we were celebrating that day. I called the three veterans who were

at the party to the front of the group and seated them in places of honor. Then we sang *God Bless America* and saluted them, which meant a lot to your Dad. Your Dad sacrificed a lot for his country. He bore a lot of physical and emotional scars from the war. Those scars are what I thought of last night when I saw the flag draped across his coffin.

I learned more about your Dad's struggles after the war when I visited him in the hospital last week. He wasn't taking any painkillers for his pain. He said he wouldn't have anything to do with morphine. Then, he told me the story of how he had become addicted to it with his injuries during the war.[4] He said that there weren't facilities during wartime for fixing the injury. Instead, he said the soldiers were "doped up" until medical services could be provided. After being on morphine for many months, he got hooked on it. After his injuries were repaired and healed, he continued on the morphine. He told me about a time when he beat up a pharmacist friend of his to get more. He said that was about the "stupidest" thing he ever did and was deeply ashamed, but it served as the wake-up call to kick his habit. He kicked it the only way he knew how. He went off into a cabin in the woods. He stayed there by himself and sweated it out. Your Dad said it was pure hell. He sat with a loaded gun to his head and his finger on the trigger for many of those days. I think it was a combination of will power on your Dad's part, defiance toward his father, and faith in God that kept him from pulling that trigger. At any rate, as I listened to your Dad's story, my respect for him deepened. I had a greater appreciation of his stoicism. I had a deeper sense of who he was and why he was.

Your Dad had a hard life. And I think these last 10 years after he retired enabled him to let the grizzly bear in him fade and the tender teddy bear emerge. These were years when your Dad softened with age so that insight and wisdom grew, and pride and introver-

sion faded, years that softened the blows in life that your
Dad had to face and the hardness that it took for him
to face them. My hope is that through his death, you
will have a deeper sense of his life, a deeper sense of his
love for you, and a deeper sense of yourselves.

Bereavement with Veterans

Stoicism sometimes interferes with veterans' willingness to receive bereavement services. They might fear being a "cry baby," losing control, or becoming vulnerable. Bereavement groups are sometimes viewed as a "pity party,"
something they do not want. Thus, private counseling or coaching family
members on how to support the veteran's grief processes may be more effective.

In combat, there was no time to mourn the death of comrades; soldiers
had to keep moving or they would be killed. With grief on hold, their
bereavement needs may stagnate, but facing their own death decades later or
the death of a loved one can trigger PTSD or activate grief. Past losses during combat were often mutilating or guilt-laden.

Veterans may be aware that they have unresolved grief. This awareness
can cause a fear of grieving when a member of their own family dies. "If I
start crying, I may not be able to stop." It's helpful for them see that this is
an opportunity to go back and grieve what they were not able to grieve at
the time. However, this may need to be done later, so that it doesn't interfere with their current grief work.

For veterans who have served in dangerous assignments, their past
experiences with death might have been violent and mutilating. They bring
this experience with them whenever they encounter death or grief. I try to
help them distinguish their past experiences from their current experience so
that they can encounter death peacefully.

It's often helpful to place two veterans together in the same room when
they are receiving hospice or palliative care. There is great camaraderie as
they care for each other. Grief can also be facilitated as staff help them grieve
their roommate's death. Seeing the respect with which their roommate is
treated and also how peacefully they died, can also allay the veterans' fears
about their own death.

If the veteran has PTSD, he/she probably doesn't trust easily or is reti-
cent to reach out to strangers trying to provide bereavement care. They

might cope with grief by isolating or "bunkering down," which is often counterproductive. Initial approaches by others may need to be modified and should focus on gaining trust.

On the other hand, the brother/sisterhood that saw veterans through dangerous times is often called into action when their buddy is dying. They come to bedside to care for their falling comrade. Afterward, they often check on their fallen comrade's family to make sure their needs are being met.

Stoicism, PTSD, or alcohol abuse might create multiple family estrangement, or forgiveness issues. Any of these can complicate peaceful dying and effective grieving.

Exacerbation of mental illness can occur when there is a death in the family. Bereavement programs need to be an integral part of psychiatric programs for veterans.

Veterans might feel angry or bitter about medals they didn't receive, service-connected disabilities the didn't get, pensions they didn't receive, or agent orange damage that went unacknowledged. This situation sometimes shields them from effectively encountering their need for grieving.

Veterans, who are receiving a pension that ends with their death, might fight hard to stay alive for financial purposes. Concern about their spouse's welfare might cause them to want futile medical treatments. This focus sometimes interferes with anticipatory grieving for their own life, and it prevents essential dialogue with family members which subsequently complicates their bereavement.

Military funerals include presenting an American flag to a family member. If there are disputes within families or if there has been divorce with multiple blended families, issues surrounding "Who gets the flag?" might arise. The resulting anger can complicate bereavement.

Veterans are eligible for free burial at a national cemetery, as well as their spouses. This sometimes eases financial burdens, facilitating "good grief."

The author wishes to acknowledge the contributions of Pat McGuire, Bereavement Coordinator at Bay Pines VA, for her collaboration in developing the unique considerations for providing bereavement care to veterans and their families.

Rituals for Use with PTSD[1]

This appendix chronicles rituals that were used by the West Haven, Connecticut, VA to facilitate recovery and healing from trauma. The ritual ceremonies are used at different points in the six-week inpatient treatment program. (See chapter 5 for the transition ritual used in the middle of the West Haven program.) This appendix includes the opening and closing rituals done with the family, as well as a bereavement ritual to facilitate grieving for fallen comrades.

This first ritual is the opening ceremony the West Haven VA uses with veterans who have PTSD. The families accompany the veterans to the facility and release them for treatment with this ceremony:

> **Leader:** As a country we sent you to war a long time ago and you have not fully returned to us. We the staff have been directed by the President, the Congress, the Veterans Administration to create a program that will help you come home to your families and loved ones at last.
> **Staff:** We have been sent to find you and bring you back.
> **Leader:** You, the family and friends of these veterans have had to put up with the worry, troubles, and pain of PTSD (an illness of misunderstanding, anger, memory) all these years because a country has turned its back on these men and women. Before we can accept them fully into the program, we need and they need your blessing to release them to us. Are you willing to release them to us?
> **Families:** Yes. We are willing.
> (Each veteran and his family are then asked to stand up as their name is called. Each are addressed individually.)
> **Leader:** (Calling each veteran by name, one at a time)

Mr. _____ do you want to come home from _____
(Vietnam, Korea, World War II arena where served)?
Veteran: Yes I do.
Families: We give our blessing because we love you and
we want you to come home to us.
(Veteran says goodbye to his family with a hug or hand-
shake and walks across the room to the staff.)
Leader: Veterans, are you willing to enter this program
knowing you will face the risks of change?
Veterans: Yes we are willing.
Leader: Are you willing to examine your past behaviors
toward your loved ones: the cutting off, the dumping,
the isolation, in order to regain some of the strength,
the love, and the passion that still remains in your relationships?
Veterans: Yes we are.
Leader: Family and friends of these veterans, do you
realize they are suffering from a chronic condition for
which they are not to blame?
Families: We are learning this.
Leader: Do you realize you too have suffered as a result
of their illness?
Families: Yes, we have suffered too.
Leader: Are you willing to accept their progress in small
steps?
Families: Yes, we are.
Leader: Are you willing to examine your own behavior
and make changes where necessary to allow them to
come home and resume a more responsible role?
Families: Yes, we are willing.
Leader: (To everyone) Are you all willing to fight
against the deadly voices of hopelessness, shaming,
blaming, and revenge?
Everyone: Yes, we will not listen to these voices.
Leader: Will you reach for acceptance of the bad things
that have happened, let go of the blame for suffering
from PTSD, and open yourself toward forgiveness of
others and yourself?

Everyone: Yes. We will.
Leader: (After all the veterans have lined up behind him) We have found these veterans. Now the journey home begins. (The veterans and the staff exit the room.)

The end of the program six weeks later is marked with a ceremony that returns each veteran to family and friends:

Leader: Are those gathered here willing to be witnesses for this combat veteran?
Audience: Yes we are.
Leader: (Leader turns to each veteran in turn and asks these questions. Each gives his own answers.) Did you serve our country in war? When was your tour of duty? In so doing, did you put your life at risk? Did you see death, stupidity, fear, or cowardice? Did you see courage, love, and heroism?
Audience: That is war.
Leader: Did you do things you regret? That you were proud of? Did you have experiences that are beyond words?
Audience: That is war.
Leader: When you returned home were you properly debriefed? Were you ignored, stigmatized, or ridiculed?
Audience: We let you down.
Leader: Were you ever accepted as you were, a soldier who did his duty the best way you could?
Audience: We let you down.
Leader: How did this welcome affect you? As a result of the war and this welcome, did you resort to cutting off the people you love? Resort to drugs or alcohol to silence the pain? Lose control of your anger and hurt people you love? Thought about suicide as a way of ending it all? Is there still hope?
Audience: Yes, we believe there is hope.
Leader: Even though you will live with the memories of the war forever?
Audience: Yes

Leader: Even though these things happened and there is no way to change history?

Audience: Yes

Leader: Are you willing to accept yourself as you were, as a soldier who did your duty the best way you could? Are you willing to gain better control over your anger, and show your love more openly? Are you ready to work toward forgiveness of yourself and your loved ones?

Audience: We are ready to forgive you.

Leader: Even though you carry this heavy burden from the past, can you still love your family and friends? Can you still search for meaning in your life? Can you build a new future in which you can be a contributing member of society?

Audience: Yes, you can do these things.

Leader: Despite the obstacles, do you want to return to us here in the world?

Audience: Come home to us.

Leader: Veteran, please tell your family how you feel. (Each says something to the effect of: "When I entered this program I thought this was my last chance before I lost you and the kids. I'm amazed you have been there for me through everything I have done. I promise you there will be no more abuse. I promise you I will do my best, even though I'm going to need your support more than ever with my illness. I want to be with you. I am so sorry for everything. I do love you.")

Leader: Now make the crossing.

(Leader shakes the veteran's hand and then the vet walks across the room to his family/friends as the audience breaks into applause.)

At the end of the ceremony, the leader says: "These few steps across the room are only symbolic ones, for it is not so easy to come home from war. It has affected us all and together we must work hard not to fall victim to the hopelessness and despair that beset us. I'm glad to say that tonight, at least, we have not failed."

Survivor's guilt is common for people who have experienced war or other disasters. The West Haven, Connecticut, VA developed a ritual for veterans who struggle with survivor's guilt. Staff and veterans gather at a Veteran's Memorial Park. Each veteran participant prepares a letter or other remembrance for each dead soldier held captive by the veteran's guilt. I can easily imagine the power of the ceremony:

> Leader: We come here to honor those who died in war serving their country as well as those who live and are now in mourning for them.
>
> (A wreath is ceremonially placed with each person placing a small flag or flower in it.)
>
> Leader: Oh, veterans, you men and women with the burden of dead souls captured in battle when God was not around, it's time to let these dead souls go. Place them in God's hands. Now you can mourn their death and the death of your own youth and innocence. Then you can remember.
>
> Staff: Let them go and then you can be comforted.
>
> Leader: Release them to the air, to the sea, to the earth, and let them rest at last.
>
> Staff: To the air, the sea, and the earth.
>
> Veterans: As a survivor of war, I have witnessed the deaths of men and women I loved.
>
> Staff: We know you have.
>
> Veterans: As a survivor of war, I have taken into my keeping the souls of these dead soldiers. It was my choice.
>
> Staff: A fateful choice.
>
> Veterans: As a survivor of war, this has been my sacred responsibility, to carry the memory of the dead. This responsibility has been both a burden and a solace.
>
> Staff: You have fulfilled your responsibility.
>
> Veterans: I have not betrayed or forgotten the memory of the dead.
>
> Staff: You have honored the dead.
>
> Veterans: This understanding has changed my life forever for better and for worse.
>
> Staff: For better and for worse.

Leader: Let these spirits give you inspiration and guidance for the rest of your lives. It is time for them to release you to your future. We must ask their blessing.

Veterans: Dear comrades, you will always inspire me to do my best. I need your blessing in order to go on with my life. I need your love now more than ever. Will you release me to the world?

Leader: Listen! They are with us. (Long silence) It is now time to release the souls of the dead to God, to the Earth, and to us. Please come forward and place their names in the chalice.

Staff: We know of your sadness. Tell us their names.

(Each veteran comes forward and puts the paper into the chalice and says the name out loud. Everyone repeats each name.)

Veterans: Dear comrades, I give you up to the Earth and to God. I will remember you always. Now it is time to rest.

Leader: (lighting the chalice) You, the living men and women of war, have carried this burden for more than 20 years. At this moment your unshed tears are seen. We can't change the past, but we will be with you into the future. This is our pledge. Now we commit you, dear dead comrades, to the air.

Veterans: These men and women deserve to be honored.

Staff: We honor the lives and deaths of these men and women.

Veterans: These soldiers died for their country.

Staff: We remember they died for their country.

Veterans: We commit them to the air.

Leader: In so doing, we say farewell comrades until we meet again.

All: Farewell, comrades, until we meet again.

Leader: Sing me a farewell song. A canticle of life,
For I am leaving land, and taking space to life
Into the rising wind, I'll shout the ecstasy
Echoes will answer back, I am where I wished to be.

(There is a long silence as the papers burn and the smoke goes up into the sky. The leader leads the group down to a nearby body of water.)

Leader: We now commit you to the sea.

(The leader then throws a handful of sand from another pot into the water. Each person then comes forward to scatter these ashes into the sea. Then the group returns to a place near the memorial and forms a large circle).

Leader: We now commit you to the earth.

(A veteran digs a hole in the ground. Another veteran places the ashes from the chalice in the ground and plants flowers over them. Everyone holds hands.)

Leader: May these souls find peace and be at home in the universe. May they be blessed and honored forever. May we, the living, remember them always as we turn from this place and return to our friends and family who are waiting for us. Life is long. Let the memory of these men and women give us strength.

Appendix F

Therapeutic Rituals: A Forum for Reckoning with Change

This appendix will help readers value the therapeutic role of rituals. Once these rituals are valued, my hope is that people will then use them to navigate important changes in their lives.

The Power of Myth,[1] a book by Joseph Campbell, awakened me to the value of myths and rituals and their relationship to the change and recovery process. To my scientific mind, myths were untruths. Yet, here this brilliant professor was showing me that myths spoke truths of personhood and humankind. Just like parables (stories that are not "factual") are used because words cannot completely embody truth, so too do myths embody larger truths. Myths use symbols that access the energy of the unconscious. Campbell reminds us that truth is often hidden in symbols, requiring non-physical eyes to see.

Campbell speaks similarly about rituals. To me, the word "ritual" meant a habit that was empty of meaning, robotical, automatic, habitual. However, Campbell writes that the rituals to which he speaks are just the opposite. They are filled with meanings that provide maps for navigating change. They provide order in the midst of chaos. Just as myths speak a larger truth of the unconscious, so do rituals. For healing to be complete and heartfelt, the unconscious mind must be engaged. Rituals provide access to energy of the unconscious.

The term "ritual" often has a negative connotation; people sometime associate it with cults or gangs. Unsavory groups do take advantage of ritualized forums, but they also use other forums such as speech and books to disseminate their message. Yet, the rest of us don't stop speaking or reading for fear it might link us to something sinister; neither should we fear rituals. In fact, the more I learned about rituals, the more convinced I became of their therapeutic value. The more I let go of my preconceived ideas about what I thought rituals were, the more I became open to their effectiveness in reckoning with change. I realized that in times of uncertainty, loss, and

225

change, therapeutic rituals provided a format for letting go of the old, integrating the uncertainty of change, and redefining a hopeful future. I became so convinced of their value that in graduate school, I designed my master's thesis on the relationship between rituals and hope. I embarked carefully upon the study of designing therapeutic rituals that could be used clinically to provide support, guidance, and hope for hospice patients and families as they faced the uncertainty of changes that accompany death.

In my study of therapeutic ritual, I learned the importance of choosing symbols for rituals that have shared meanings for the individual or within the group. I also learned about the three stages of ritual: separation, transition, and integration.

Separation Stage

The purpose of this stage is to acknowledge difficulties that make change necessary and to recognize the need to separate from former roles or identities. During this stage, there is a request to reframe unwanted change into a *desire* to change. Military rituals are formatted with highly evocative styles and symbols. Patriotic music and American flags activate unconscious images that motivate new identity and new will. Induction rituals help new recruits separate from civilian identity. Uniforms are issued; heads shaved. Recruits are sometimes ridiculed for their former immature, lazy, and civilian ways.

Many religious rituals might begin with a confession of sinfulness or ways we separate ourselves from God. Funeral rites or memorial services start with the acknowledgement of death and the hope for facing life without the loved one. In the ritual with Paul (Chapter 5), we started with an acknowledgment of war deeds for which he felt remorseful.

The separation stage is crucial in creating an effective ritual. In a grief-denying, "never say good-bye" culture, it's tempting to skip to the integration stage without giving adequate time and energy to articulating the need for change and separation. If the need for change is not openly expressed, the silence reinforces fear of the problem, heightening the control it exerts. The whole point of a therapeutic ritual is to create a safe environment whereby the problem can emerge from hiding so its power can be diminished and the person's empowerment to deal with the problem can be enhanced.

Transition Stage

This stage is often the turning point for acceptance or rejection of the change that is being offered. Anxiety or resistance can be anticipated to be highest at this stage. Participants are asked to leave behind the familiar and antici-pate a new beginning without knowing what that will mean. Old identities are let go while new identities are not yet secured. Straddling two worlds, people don't feel like they yet belong to either.

In the military, the transition stage is used to indoctrinate recruits with a basic training that promotes warrior perspectives. The transition stage in religious rites might include readings or sermons that encourage change and living a more godly life. Funeral rites eulogize the deceased person during this transition stage of the burial ritual. In Paul's service, Chaplain Dan told the story of the prodigal son, and the Vietnam veteran volunteer told his own story of recovery from war. Stories en-courage people to let go of past brokenness and open up to hope for a different future.

Integration Stage

The final stage of a therapeutic ritual is integration. This stage seeks to instill hope for a future that promises growth. Thus, the ceremony is closed with a sense of renewal and confidence that change can be navigated. A symbol is often given that participants can take home with them. They are encouraged to let the symbol act as an inspiration to continue with the change.

In the military, the integration phase culminates at the end of basic training with graduation ceremonies that symbolize the new warrior identi-ty. In religious services, this phase might include celebration rites such as communion. In funeral rites, it might include a challenge to let the deceased person's admirable qualities inspire others or assist in filling the gap the per-son leaves behind. In Paul's service, the integration phase included his abso-lution by the priest, being welcomed into the folds of the team with a group hug, and team members telling him the impact his story had made on us.

With rituals, it's tempting to convey that the broken past is no more, but the goal is not to remove a painful past which would only serve to rein-force denial or other flighting behaviors. The goal is to develop a different relationship to the past and instill confidence that the participant(s) can cope with the past in a new way that gives their future new meaning. It encour-ages participants to redeem their suffering with new insight from lessons learned.

The stages of ritual also correspond to how we interpret time: past, present, and future. The first stage of a ritual (separation phase) reflects a new willingness to abide with the past, acknowledging the specific broken-ness that was incurred. The next stage (transition) highlights the present, where a releasing of the past is done and there is a reckoning with the uncer-tainty and ambiguities of the present. The last stage of integration expresses a decision that beholds hope for a different future. Campbell's book, *The Hero with a Thousand Faces*,[2] describes how this format depicts the timeless journey all of us are required to make if we are to become heroes in our own lives.

Rituals to Navigate Unwanted Change

I have used rituals professionally when difficult transitions were needed. When our oncology unit developed the hospice program, we didn't antici-pate the strife and division it would cause staff. Creation of new programs with different patients upset the usual pattern of care. Tension and argu-ments ensued as staff coped with the change. Staff were reluctant to let go of their identity as oncology nurses and expand into the identity of oncology and hospice nurses. The new identity was necessary for the unit to function successfully.

I designed a therapeutic ritual to promote the inward changes needed to incorporate the larger identity that was needed. During the separation stage of the ritual, each staff member recalled a cherished memory, said good-bye to "the good old days," and acknowledged the difficulty and pain of doing so. Each proclaimed a desire to grow into a new identity that included hospice nursing. Each brought spiritual readings and songs that reflected letting go and saying good-bye. During the transition stage, the anxiety of journeying into unfamiliar territory was acknowledged. Songs and readings that reflected a willingness to stay open to the uncertainty were articulated, as well as a willingness to suffer required changes. Each person acknowledged the difficulty of changing and identified something they needed to do in order to make the transition into hospice nursing. A circle was formed with each person lighting a candle, saying, "A heart that is will-ing to suffer is a light to the world." The integration stage included receiv-ing a small footprints pin with the words, "Know that your journey is sacred and that your footprints are holy." Songs that appealed to the hope of living from our larger selves were sung; a final blessing dispensed.

There were many tears during this ceremony. There was also much change. There was no longer a need to fight or resist. Problems still arose, but they were dealt with openly and with understanding. I subsequently modified the ritual and used it at the conclusion of each "Living and Dying Healed" course I teach.

Therapeutic Rituals Surrounding Illness and Death

Rituals are enacted at time of death on our Hospice and Palliative Care unit. These rituals are especially important in our underritualized, death-denying, "we-don't-need-a-funeral" culture. A flag replaces the blanket on the bed while family have time with their loved one's body. The body is then transported to the morgue under the flag. As it passes down the hallway, people often stand aside and pay respect with a salute. The patient is also honored by placing on the bed a rose and footprint with his/her name and date of death. The six-inch footprints are made by staff from baked dough that is molded into the shape of footprints. When the dough hardens, it is painted.

This footprint honors the veteran and also highlight his separation from us. Other patients see the footprint and anticipate that they, too, will be remembered and treated with respect. This footprint also acts as a trigger in the environment for them to anticipate and prepare for their own deaths. The footprint remains on the bed until another patient comes to occupy the bed. Then it's moved to a wall in the hallway that depicts a rainbowed road with the inscription, "Together we walk, one step at a time." (See Chapter 7 for a picture of the wall.) The wall with all the collected footprints acts as another trigger in the environment for death preparation. In November, the footprint is moved to a holiday tree and later given back to the family members at a holiday bereavement program.

Another important ritual occurs with the family at time of death. After a loved one's death, an electric candle is lit with the family. The pain they are feeling is acknowledged. The courage to let go is affirmed. Family members are en-couraged to tell a few of their favorite stories about their loved one. Each is then asked to write a message to their loved one on the back of the patient's name card, one more opportunity to address "unfinished business." The card is placed on a stand in front of the candle. A prayer or reading that offers hope and support for continuing without the loved one is provided. Marianne Williamson's book of spiritual prayers, *Illuminata*,[3] is often used.

It has one section devoted to prayers for use in therapeutic rituals. A pin with three footprints is then pinned on each person with staff providing a message of hope. "One footprint is yours. One footprint is your loved one's. The third footprint represents all the people who are willing to help you walk this painful part of your journey. May each time you see these, you know you are not alone. May you have the courage to ask for help when you need it." As modern culture continues to devalue grief, as mourning is shortened from months to days, and as funeral services are eliminated, this ritual becomes increasingly valued.

The Grief Recovery group also uses rituals to process grief. Bereaved group members finger paint a picture that reminds them of their loved one. One by one, they light a candle and explain the picture to the group. They also tell their loved one whatever they want them to know or speak any unfinished business. Then they blow the candle out, while being affirmed that they can meet the challenges of a new world without their loved one in it.

We use ritualized formats that incorporate the three stages of change for several bereavement events. We hold a Memorial service every four months to honor all the veterans who died in the Medical Center. On Memorial Day, we use a ritualized format to provide bereavement care at a picnic. All of these rituals are well attended with more than 200 family members in attendance.

When employees die, especially if it's an unexpected death that leaves unfinished business, I meet with the employees on that unit. A candle is lit, a memorial card with the person's name and date of death is given to each person. They write their good-byes on it during the opening separation stage. During the transition phase, a picture or some other object is passed and each person recalls a story about the deceased person. In the integration phase, each person identifies one quality of the deceased they are willing to let inspire them.

We use a ritualized format for other processes: Quality of Life gatherings, presenting veteran certificates and pins, gracious receiver buttons, and Native American talking-stick[4] sessions with staff. I often try to ritualize ordinary processes. For example, volunteers make lap blankets; they leave them with the staff to give to the patients. Now, we have them write a note about why they made the blanket for them and we present it to the patient, acknowledging the difficulties they are having and presenting them with a symbol of care and support. There's a dramatic difference in the impact of the blanket depending on whether or not the presentation is ritualized.

I use the ritualized format when I do guided imagery with patients. Rather than only visualizing a finished product (for example, an improved relationship), I have patients imagine the process: communicating the problem clearly and without blame (separation from old patterns); opening up to hear the other person and projecting self into the other person imagining how they think, feel, and want to communicate (transitioning into give and take tension of a changing relationship); and imagining accepting the other person's position, whatever it is, without closing off to their personhood so that a new relationship can be born (integration stage).

I also used ritualized formats in counseling sessions and in personal circumstances surrounding loss and change. A loss by death might prompt a written message or letter to give voice to unspoken fears, guilt, anger, and longing. I might encourage the person to read the message at graveside, send the letter on the tail of a helium balloon, or ignite the letter so it goes up in flames. These enactments add further symbolic value that reaches into the unconscious for deeper healing.

The loss of a marriage might prompt enactment of a ritual surrounding the removal of a wedding ring along with hope for successfully suffering the changes that will be forthcoming. Successfully suffering a divorce can grow a person into their larger self just as unsuccessfully suffering divorce can reduce a person into smallness that hardens and embitters their heart with fear and pain.

My friends and I have begun birthday ritual adventures that humorously welcome us into "crone-ism." It helps us resist the urge to protest our aging. Instead, we open up to its redemptive blessings by valuing the lesson of humility that aging teaches, unless it's bypassed with a facelift. As my 90-year-old mother tells me, "It takes a lot of courage to grow old."

Appendix G

Life Review

This appendix provides an example of a Life Review form that our Hospice and Palliative Care unit uses to assist in the healing process. There are two forms. One is for the patient to complete on him/herself with family/friend assistance. I tell people to just ask the questions and get the patient talking while the family/friend jots down some of the responses. It's not so much about completing the form; rather, it's about sharing the stories. The other form is for the patient to complete on other family members and also for family members to complete on the patient. I encourage them to consider mailing Life Review forms to family members unable to be present at this time. I also encourage them to come together as a group and share what each has written. This meeting can be a very powerful and meaningful time together. It is a time of recalling stories and sharing them with each other, a final gift that often creates tears, laughter, and cherished memories.

I also tell them to consider writing letters to family members that could be given to them after their death. For example, if they will miss a child's graduation, wedding, etc., they can write a letter to them expressing their hopes. It's a way they can be non-physically present that day. They then give the letter to someone who can give it to their loved one on the occasion. Another alternative is to complete a Life Review form on each young family member so it can be given to them when they grow older. They will then know the meaning they had in the dying person's life, which helps give them a deeper sense of themselves.

I encourage them to take every opportunity to enhance the meaningfulness of this precious time in their family's life. These forms can help do that. The forms also become precious keepsakes after a loved one's death and can also provide a meaningful basis for developing a eulogy or other tribute.

Life Review: Self
(Patient to respond with family writing responses)

One of my favorite childhood memories is:

_____

_____

_____

Words that describe me include:

_____

_____

_____

One way in which my military service impacted my life is:

_____

_____

_____

One of the most difficult things for me to deal with in my lifetime has been:

_____

_____

_____

The reason this was so difficult was because:

_____

_____

_____

What I have learned because of the burdens I have endured is:

_____

_____

_____

One of the things I am most proud of is:

_____

_____

One of the things I like best about myself is:

_____

_____

If I were to live my life over again, something I would change is:

_____

_____

If I were to live my life over again, something I would not change is:

_____

_____

One of the ways I think I have touched other peoples' lives is:

_____

_____

One of the things I most want to be remembered for is:

_____

_____

If I could give one piece of advice to someone it would be:

_____

_____

Something that would bring me more peace right now is:

_____

_____

_____

Something I want to say to my family/friends is:

_____

_____

_____

Life Review
(Patient to complete on others)
(Family/friends to complete on patient)

My favorite story about my loved one is:

_____

_____

A memory that will always make me laugh is:

_____

_____

A favorite story from my childhood about my loved one is:

_____

_____

A meaningful story my loved one told me about his/her childhood is:

_____

_____

_____

A story from the military my loved one has told me that I'll never forget is:

_____

_____

One of the things I most appreciate about my loved one is:

_____

_____

One way in which my loved one has touched my life is:

_____

_____

The difference this has made for my life is:

_____

_____

A virtue that my loved one has that I want to carry on in my own life is:

_____

_____

Something I think would bring my loved one more peace right now is:

_____

_____

A hope I have for my loved one right now is:

_____

_____

_____

Something I want to say to my loved one is:

_____

_____

_____

Appendix H

Resources

Veterans Families United Foundation (405-535-1925) www.VeteransFamiliesUnited.org. Helps veterans and their families cope with the aftermath of war and provides information about accessing benefits.

Military One Source (1-800-342-9647) www.militaryonesource.com. Provides counselors 24 hours/day.

National Center for Posttraumatic Stress Disorder. www.ncptsd.va.gov. Provides information about PTSD.

National Alliance on Mental Illness (NAMI) www.nami.org/veterans. Describes various mental health issues affecting veterans.

America Supports You www.americasupportsyou.mil. A Department of Defense website that connects veterans with organizations willing to provide services.

Vet Centers (1-800-905-4675;1-866-496-8838) www.vetcenter.va.gov. Provides readjustment counseling and outreach services to all veterans who served in any combat zone, as well as services for their family members for military-related issues. Services are provided at no cost. There are 232 community-based Vet Centers located in all fifty states.

Department of Veterans Affairs, Veteran Recovery www.veteranrecovery.med.va.gov. A Vet-to-Vet peer support program to provide mutual support in recovery.

www.goldstarmom.com. Support for mothers who have had a child killed in the military.

www.goldstarwives.org. Support for wives who have had husbands killed in the military.

www.nhpco.org/veterans. Scroll down to "Helpful Resources." Click on
"VA Transforms End-of-Life Care for Veterans."

www.nhpco.org. search: veterans. The National Hospice and Palliative
Care website provides numerous articles, books, and tool kits to provide
end-of-life care for veterans.

www.tidewell.org. (800-959-4291). This hospice has an inspirational
"Honors Program" that includes: a recognition ceremony for veterans, leaving a veteran legacy program, and a pinning for families caring for veterans. Additionally, they provide support groups and bereavement groups for
families of soldiers and veterans.

Hospice of Case Western Reserve in Cleveland Ohio offers an outstanding
program for veterans entitled, Peaceful and Proud. Reference this program
at www.hospicewr.org.

Denise DiGiovanni-Segal at Vitas Innovative Hospice Care of the Palm
Beaches (561- 364-1479). This nurse is a role-model for providing hospice
services to veterans, as well as partnering with VA medical centers to assure
care. Go to www.palmbeachpost.com, to read about her work: "Hospice
Worker Makes sure Dying Veterans Get Their Due." May 21, 2008.

This book can be be a powerful resource for healing veterans. Give it to
one. Even better, give a copy to someone who loves a veteran. If you are an
organization or agency who deals with veterans, consider using this book as
a fund raiser. Contact the author on her website:
www.deborahgrassman.com to learn how to do this. Also, many veteran
organizations such as the American Legion, Veterans of Foreign Wars, and
Disabled American Veteran organizations are often willing to fund projects
for veterans.

Endnotes

Chapter One
[1] Deborah Grassman
[2] VA photographs taken by Tim Westmorland.
[3] www.va.gov/visn8/baypines/aboutus/history
[4] Grassman, D. (1993) Oncology Nursing Forum. Development of Oncology Educational and Support Programs. Vol. 20 (4). 669-676.
[5] The word *palliate* means "to soothe." When quantity of life can no longer be controlled, palliative care focuses on quality of life with comfort and symptom management as the priority. Hospice is a subspecialty of palliative care geared toward people who are nearing the end of their lives. In addition to aggressive pain and symptom control, hospice care focuses on emotional and spiritual preparation for reckoning with end-of-life issues. The goal of hospice is to help people die healed.

Chapter Two
[1] *Romeo and Juliet*
[2] Real name used with permission of Tommy Bills. To contact Tommy, e-mail him at 1stcav@wildblue.com.
[3] See Appendix A for Tommy's complete diary, as well as my response. This appendix also includes poems written by women who served in the Vietnam War. Like Tommy, they used the arts to help recover from Posttraumatic Stress Disorder (PTSD).
[4] For further information about the artist and the Veteran's Day Display, see article by J. Sanders, entitled "Vietnam Veteran's Paintings Draw out Long-denied Feelings" in the *St. Petersburg Times,* November 16, 1993 (retrieve on-line via archives at www.stpetetimes.com).

Chapter Three
[1] May, Rollo (1969). *Love and Will.* NY: Dell, p. 263, 292.
[2] Statistics cited by Scott Shreve DO, Chief of Hospice and Palliative Care Services for the Department of Veterans Affairs. Connecticut Healthcare System Annual Conference on Hospice and Palliative Care. October 28, 2008.
[3] I'm indebted to Joseph Zanchelli who wrote me about how military culture interfered with his civilian life after he was discharged from service.

I've selected some of his quotes that typify those I've heard from other veterans. I've added other quotes not cited by Zanchelli that I've heard from multiple other veterans. The quotes can not be generalized to every veteran's experience.

[4] For an enlightening perspective on the difficulty of returning to civilian life, read "The Price of Valor" by Dan Baum in *The New Yorker*, July 12, 2004, available online. See excerpts of the article in Chapter 5.

[5] *Webster's New World Dictionary* (1995). NY: Simon & Schuster

[6] See Appendix B for interactions that help create a safe emotional space that can respond to stoicism.

[7] Grossman, D. (1996). *On Killing: The Psychological Cost of Learning to Kill in War and Society.* NY: Little Brown and Co., p. 260.

Chapter Four

[1] *Looming* by Karl Michaud. National Vietnam Veterans Art Museum. Chicago.

[2] Dale Sameulson, artist.

[3] Chemical warfare with Agent Orange defoliant was being used by American soldiers against the Vietnamese. Years later, when soldiers started experiencing effects from Agent Orange, the government disregarded their complaints. Vets had to organize and fight to receive attention, treatment, and compensation.

[4] Viktor Frankl, a concentration camp survivor put it: "The crowning experience for the homecoming man is the wonderful feeling that, after all he has suffered, there is nothing he need fear any more—except his God." *Man's Search for Meaning* (1984). NY: Washington Square Press, p. 115.

[5] For more information about the mythical story *The Crescent Moon Bear*, see Chapter 7 or read *Women Who Run with the Wolves* by Clarissa Pinkola Estes.

[6] This patient's real name, Milton Howarth, is being used with permission of his sister, Ester Howarth. Tearfully, she speaks of how Milton's artistic spirit sensitized him to the horror of war. She also showed me a book of sketches about camplife that Milton had drawn in the dark of night, hiding them under his shirt. Milton's obituary can be found in the *St. Petersburg Times*, Oct. 23, 2003, available on-line.

[7] Pueschel M. PTSD prevention, care techniques debated. *US Medicine* 2004; 40(4):1-24.

[8] *Diagnostic And Statistical Manual Of Mental Disorders,* 4th ed. (2000). Washington, D.C: APA, p. 467-468.

[9] See Appendix C for more information about PTSD.

[10] When used in these kinds of situations, fine is said to be an acronym for: freaked-out, insecure, neurotic, and emotional.

[11] This patient's real name, Ed Chaffin, is being used with his permission.

[12] See Appendix D for more information about unique considerations for providing bereavement care to veterans and also to their families.

[13] The chaplain's name is Mike Neal at Tidewell Hospice serving Sarasota and the surrounding Florida counties. Tidewell has an HONORS program that includes caring for families of veterans, families of those currently in the military, and families who have lost an active service member or veteran. They partner with the Red Cross and other agencies to provide services. Their program also includes a legacy project in which a veteran's service story is recorded. To acknowledge veterans, they have a team of volunteers who are veterans that go to the patient's home to pin him/her and present a certificate of appreciation. For more information, go to www.tidewell.org.

[14] Department of Defense and Veterans Administration websites.

[15] Read the book of Job, especially chapter seven. It describes Job's response to the trauma of losing his children, wealth, and health. For further reading about Job, see Jung, CG. (1958). *Answer to Job.* Princeton: Princeton University Press.

[16] "VA must offer to provide or purchase hospice & palliative care that VA determines an enrolled veteran needs" (38 CFR 17.36 and 17.38).

[17] *St.Petersburg Times.* April 22, 2005. Opinion section. Available online at www.stpetetimes.com

[18] *Diagnostic And Statistical Manual Of Mental Disorders,* 4th ed. (2000). Washington, D.C: APA, p. 467-468.

[19] www.vetcenter.va.gov for more information.

[20] Vrana S, Lauterbach D: Prevalence of traumatic events and post-traumatic psychological symptoms in a nonclinical sample of college students. *J. Traumatic Stress.* 1994; 289-302.

Chapter Five

[1] Van Devanter L, Furey JA ed. (1991). *Visions of War, Dreams of Peace.* NY: Warner Books, p. 149. See Appendix A for writings by women who suffered PTSD from the Vietnam War. The poems helped them abide

and reckon with their memories so they could recover.

[2] Her real name, Memrie Wilkes, is being used with permission of her nephew, John Wilkes.

[3] Holm, Jeanne (1998). *In Defense of Nation: Servicewomen in World War II*. St. Petersburg, FL: Vandamere Press.

[4] Ormerod, AJ, Fitzgerald, LF, Collinsworth, LL, Lawson, AK, Lytell, M, Perry, LA, Wright, CV. (2006). *Sexual Assault in the Military: Context Factors and Measurement Issues*. Urbana, Ill: University of Illinois. The range of reported assault varies from 3.3%-23%. The actual incidence of assault is difficult to know since only 15%-25% of victims report its occurrence. One study of 558 Vietnam and Gulf War female veterans found that 30% had been sexually assaulted. It should also be noted that though there is a higher percentage of women assaulted, there are more men sexually assaulted than women because there is a much higher proportion of men serving in the military.

[5] Baum, Dan "The Price of Valor." *The New Yorker*. July 2005.

[6] The song was *Gather*, which has lines that acknowledge our brokenness: "Gather us in the blind and the lame. Call to us now and we shall awaken. We shall arise at the sound of our name. Gather us in the rich and the haughty. Gather us in the proud and the strong. Give us a heart so meek and so lowly. Give us the courage to enter the song. Gather us in and hold us forever. Gather us in and make us your own. Gather us in all peoples together, fire of love in our flesh and our bone." Text and tune by Marty Haugen. 1982. GIA Publications, Inc.

[7] If Paul had been unwilling to provide the details of his story, we would have en-couraged him to write the details down so that his guilt could be acknowledged privately but specifically. Specificity is important.

[8] Awake and Greet the New Dawn. Text: Psalm 98; Timothy Dudley-Smith. Tune: Cantate Domino; David G. Wilson. 1973. Hope Publishing Co.

[9] *Holy Bible*. (19821982). Nashville: Thomas Nelson Inc. Luke 15: 11-32.

[10] Scott Fairchild, presenting at a PTSD conference at Wuesthoff Hospice in Brevard County, Florida, reports that there have been 14,600 wars historically.

[11] References cite varying statistics for the prevalence of suicide following the Vietnam War, ranging from 20,000 to 200,000. For more information see www.suicidewall.com. It should be noted that these suicide statistics do not include suicide-type behaviors that result in death such as

reckless driving, overdosing on drugs, etc.

[12] Johnson, DR, Feldman, SC, Lubin, H, Southwick, SM. The therapeutic use of ritual and ceremony in the treatment of posttraumatic stress disorder. *J of Traumatic Stress* 1995; 8:283-297.

[13] See Appendix E for the ceremonies used by the West Haven VA.

[14] See Appendix F for more information on the role and value of therapeutic rituals for healing.

[15] See Appendix D for more information about the unique bereavement needs of veterans.

[16] The Gold Star Mothers Club was formed after World War I to provide support for mothers who lost sons or daughters in the war. The name came from the custom of families hanging a banner in the window of their homes. The banner had a star for each family member in the military. Living servicemen were represented by a blue star, and those who had lost their lives were represented by a gold star. Gold Star Mother's Day is observed on the last Sunday in September.

Chapter Six

[1] Ron Mann, Atoning, in the National Vietnam Veterans Art Museum, Chicago.

[2] Anxious energy usually rises. Think about when you get excited. Your voice usually gets higher; energy gets flighty. You might place your hand on your chest or near your throat, involuntarily anchoring yourself. A calm, centered person's energy usually resides lower and deeper. If a calm person places their hand on an un-calm person's sternum, it can often help them feel secure, more weighted, less anxious.

[3] The name of this soldier is Richard Luttrell. To read more about his story see the *Wall Street Journal.* Jaffe, Greg. War Wounds. August 17, 2005. Mr. Luttrell's story of going to Vietnam to meet the daughter in the photo so he could ask for forgiveness was aired on May 25, 2008 on MSNBC. You can watch Keith Morrison's interview of this event on the internet: msnbc.msn.com/id/21134540/vp/24829058#24829153.

[4] See Appendix F for more information on the value of therapeutic rituals.

[5] See Appendix G for the Life Review form

[6] For further reading on the process of forgiveness and tools to accomplish it, see Flanigan, Beverly (1992). *Forgiving the Unforgivable.* NY: Macmillan.

[7] See Appendix B for interventions to facilitate forgiveness considerations.

[8] The presentation was entitled: "Sacred Conversations: The Role of Forgiveness in End-of-Life Care" by Nicholas Gross, social worker, at the 2004 Florida State Hospice Conference for Volunteers.
[9] Peck, MS. (1978). *The Road Less Traveled.* NY: Simon & Schuster.
[10] Peck, MS. (1978). *The Road Less Traveled.* NY: Simon & Schuster.
[11] The prayer is used by Alcoholics Anonymous. It is part of a longer prayer that is attributed to various sources, most commonly Reinhold Niebuhr. Though not as famous, I also like the next line of the prayer, which is: Living one day at a time; enjoying one moment at a time; accepting hardships as the pathway to peace.
[12] Remen, Rachel. (2000). *My Grandfather's Blessings.* NY: Riverhead.

Chapter Seven
[1] Cambell, Joseph (1988). *The Power of Myth.* NY: Broadway. p. 123.
[2] Cambell, Joseph (1988). *The Power of Myth.* NY: Broadway, p. 124.
[3] A *Posttraumatic Growth Inventory* scale has been developed to measure such growth and change. It includes qualities such as relating to others, new possibilities, personal strength, spiritual change, and appreciation of life. Mystakidou, K., Parpa, E., Tsilika, E., Pathiaki, M, Galanos, A., Vlahos,L. (2007). *American Journal of Hospice & Palliataive Medicine.* Traumatic distress and positive changes in advanced cancer patients. p. 270-276.
[4] Estes CP. (1992). *Women who Run with the Wolves.* NY: Random House, p. 353.
[5] Estes CP. (1992). *Women who Run with the Wolves.* NY: Random House, p. 347-350.
[6] A friend, Pat McGuire, bought me a statue for my garden: a woman with a bear headdress. "It's your trademark," she said. I look at it often and draw courage for my own journey of integrating scattered pieces of broken self into a peaceful whole by summoning the courage to meet my Crescent Moon Bear.
[7] I've noticed that many of the traditional PTSD therapies are not necessarily effective or practical in the last few days of life, especially when PTSD has not been previously diagnosed. Because the conscious mind is growing weaker in the dying, grounding people in "reality" may not be effective. It also took me a long time to distinguish the agitation and confusion of PTSD from "terminal restlessness" (a condition commonly experienced by many people the last few days of life as they transition

inward, letting go of the outer world).

[8] One of my hopes is that community hospices will start partnering with staff from Vet Centers to respond to such emergencies. Vet Centers are outreach programs for all veterans regardless of whether or not they are enrolled in the VA.

[9] Callanan M., Kelley P. (1993). *Final Gifts.* NY: Bantam Books.

[10] This patient's real name, John Bundy, is used with his permission. He knew I was writing this book. Before he died, he asked that this story be included identifying him as the source.

[11] For more information about gestalting dreams, see Perls F., Hefferline RF., Goodman P (1951) *Gestalt Therapy.* NY: Dell. For easier reading, see Perls, Frederick S. (1959). *Gestalt Therapy Verbatim.* Moab, Utah: Real People Press.

[12] Patient's real name is being used because Russell had created his manuscript in hopes that it would get published in the *St Petersburg Times* newspaper. For more details about Russell and pictures of the play, see Diggs, J. Frank (2000). *Americans Behind the Barbed Wire.* St.Petersburg, FL: Vandamere Press.

[13] *The Man Who Came to Dinner* is a comedy by George S. Kaufman and Moss Hart. It debuted in 1939 in New York City.

Chapter Eight

[1] Deborah Grassman

[2] My colleague, Tracy Thatcher, was the one who identified "going fishing" with the worms. It reminds me of Henry Nowen's book, *Wounded Healer* (1979), which allows us to use our own wounds to be a source of healing for others.

[3] VHA Directive 2003-008. (Feb. 4, 2003). Palliative care consult teams. Washington DC: Department of Veterans Affairs.

[4] Other statistics that may be relevant are: Pain intensity is significantly worse among veterans than the general public and exposure to trauma and psychological stress worsens pain and complicates effective pain treatment (American Pain Foundation. Topics in Pain Management, March 2007).

[5] For more information about the VA and NHPCO initiative to provide hospice care for veterans, see VA/NHPCO Monograph by Larry Beresford, 2005, entitled "VA Transforms End-of-Life Care for Veterans." Available on-line at

www.va.gov/oaa/archiva/ Va_Transforms_End_of_ Life_Care .pdf
and the veterans toolkit at www.nhpco/veterans.
[6] Contact the author through www.deborahgrassman.com to obtain
DVDs of *Wounded Warriors: Their Last Battle,* as well as the follow-up
DVD for training staff.

Epilogue
[1] I'm indebted to the push by my office mate, Sheila Lozier, for teaching
me Power Point, as well as medical media consultant, Rob Giles, for practical applications. They have made me computer literate . . . almost.
[2] Callanan M., Kelley P. (1993). *Final gifts.* NY: Bantam Books.
[3] Tobin, Daniel R. (1999). *Peaceful Dying.* Reading Massachusetts:
Perseus Books.
[4] Anticipate a forthcoming book on abiding, reckoning, and beholding
The Hero Within.

Appendix A
[1] Van Devanter L., Furey JA. ed. (1991). *Visions of War, Dreams of Peace.*
NY: Warner Books.

Appendix B
[1] Frey, W. (1988). Tears that Speak. *Psychology Today.* July/August, volume 18.
[2] Frankl, Viktor. (1984). *Man's Search for Meaning.* NY: Washington
Square Press.
[3] Pueschel M. PTSD prevention, care techniques debated. *US Medicine*
2004; 40(4):1-24.
[4] From presentation at Massachusetts State Hospice Conference 2006 by
the Brockton VA PTSD staff in Boston: Michele Karel Ph.D., Michael
Dodd Ph.D., and Barbara Lockwood L.C.S.W.
[5,6] For more about externalizing trauma or double listening, read publications by Michael White with Dulwich Centre Publications (www.dulwich-
centre.com.au).
[7] www.ncptsd.va.gov
[8] The first five steps: forgive me, I forgive you, I love you, Thank you,
Good-bye are from Byock, Ira (1997). *Dying Well.* NY: Riverhead Books. I
have added two more steps: Let go and open up. I believe that the reason
you do the first five steps is so you can achieve the last two.
[9] "VA must offer to provide or purchase hospice & palliative care that VA

determines an enrolled veteran needs." 38 CFR 17.36 and 17.38.

Appendix C
[1] *Diagnostic and Statistical Manual of Mental Disorders,* 4th ed. (2000). Washington, D.C.: APA,: p. 467-468.
[2] *New American Bible.* (1970) Washington DC: Job 7:13. Confraternity of Christian Doctrine. For further reading about Job, see Jung, CG. (1958) *Answers to Job.* Princeton: Princeton University Press.
[3] Pueschel M. PTSD prevention, care techniques debated. *US Medicine* 2004; 40(4):1-24.
[4] See www.ncptsd.org, www.giftfromwithin.org, www.ptsdalliance.org, www.nami.org, and www.adaa.org for more valuable information on PTSD.
[5] Epstein, J. Miller, J. *San Francisco Chronicle.* "US Wars and Post-traumatic stress disorder." June 23, 2005.
[6] Fontana, A., Rosenheck, R. (1999). A model of war zone stressors and posttraumatic stress disorder. *Journal of Traumatic Stress* 12(1): 111-126.
[7] Fontana, A., Rosenheck, R. (2004). Trauma, change in strength of religious faith, and mental health service use among veterans treated for PTSD. *Journal of Nervous and Mental Disease.* 192(9):579-584.
[8] Hoge, CW., Castro, C., Messer, S., McGurk, D., Colting, D., & Koffman, M (2004). Combat duty in Iraq and Afghanistan, mental health problems, and barriers to care. *New England Journal of Medicine* 351 (1):13-22.
[9] For insightful reading about the difference having committed violence makes, read "The Price of Valor" by Dan Baum in *The New Yorker,* July 12, 2004. See Chapter 5 for excerpts from the article.
[10] The literature also reports that PTSD causes numerous neurochemical changes in the brain. See Yehuda, R. Current concepts: post traumatic stress disorder. *New England Journal of Medicine,* 2002; 34646:108-114 Jan. 10 2002. See McEwen, Bruce S. The neurobiology and neuroendocrinology of stress, implications for post traumatic stress disorder from a basic science perspective. *Psychiatric Clinics of North America* 25 (2002) 469-494.

Appendix D
[1] Also see family considerations in Chapter 4. See Appendix E for a bereavement ritual to facilitate veterans' grief for fallen comrades.

[2] Rando, T. (1993). *Treatment of Complicated Mourning.* Champagne, Ill.: Research Press.
[3] Go to www.tidewell.org for more information about their HONORS program for veterans and their families.
[4] Taking opioids to feed an addiction should not be confused with taking opioids for end-of-life pain. Extensive research has shown that addiction to opioids taken for pain at end of life is negligible.

Appendix E
[1] Johnson, DR, Feldman, SC, Lubin, H, Southwick, SM. The therapeutic use of ritual and ceremony in the treatment of post-traumatic stress disorder. *Journal of Traumatic Stress* 1995. 8:283-297.

Appendix F
[1] Campbell, Joseph (1988). *The Power of Myth.* NY: Broadway Books.
[2] Campbell, Joseph (2004) *The Hero with a Thousand Faces.* Princeton: Princeton University Press.
[3] Williamson, Marianne (1994). *Illuminata.* NY: Random House.
[4] For more information about the therapeutic value of talking sticks, go to www.acaciart.com/stories/archive.

Index